Skin
Therapy

Cover: Fungal toe-nail infection:
(top) before treatment with terbinafine;
(middle) following 3 months' treatment
with terbinafine 250 mg per day, which
marked the end of therapy; and
(bottom) 48 weeks after the start of
therapy.

Skin Therapy

Edited by

Ronald Marks
FRCP, FRCPath
*Professor of Dermatology, University of
Wales College of Medicine, Cardiff*

and

William J. Cunliffe
MD, FRCP
*Professor of Dermatology, Leeds
Foundation for Dermatological Research*

Martin Dunitz

© Martin Dunitz Ltd 1994

First published in the United Kingdom in 1994
by Martin Dunitz Ltd, The Livery House,
7–9 Pratt Street, London NW1 0AE

A CIP catalogue record of this book is available from the
British Library.

ISBN 1-85317-138-7

Produced with an educational grant from
Sandoz Pharmaceuticals (UK) Ltd

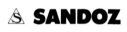

Composition by Scribe Design, Gillingham, Kent
Printed and bound in Spain

Contents

List of contributors

B. Roger Allen
Department of Dermatology, University Hospital, Queen's Medical Centre, Nottingham NG7 2UH, UK

Marcia Baum
Skin Research Foundation of California, 2001 Santa Monica Boulevard, Santa Monica, California 90404, USA

Colin B. Blakemore
Biometrics/Data Management, Shire Pharmaceutical Development Ltd, Salisbury SP1 3TS, UK

D. Anthony Burns
Department of Dermatology, Leicester Royal Infirmary, Leicester, UK

John A. Cotterill
Leeds Foundation for Dermatological Research, University of Leeds Medical School, The General Infirmary at Leeds, Great George Street, Leeds LS1 3EX, UK

William J. Cunliffe
Leeds Foundation for Dermatological Research, University of Leeds Medical School, The General Infirmary at Leeds, Great George Street, Leeds LS1 3EX, UK

Peter M. Farr
Department of Dermatology, Royal Victoria Infirmary, Newcastle upon Tyne NE1 4LP, UK

Carolyn Faulder
Longtown, Herefordshire HR2 0LD, UK

Andrew Y. Finlay
Department of Dermatology, University of Wales College of Medicine, Heath Park, Cardiff CF4 4XN, UK

Lionel Fry
Department of Dermatology, St Mary's Hospital, Praed Street, London W2 1NY, UK

John Harper
Department of Dermatology, The Hospital for Sick Children, Great Ormond Street, London WC1N 3JH, UK

Roderick J. Hay
St John's Institute of Dermatology, Guy's Hospital, London SE1 9RT, UK

Andrew Herxheimer
Cochrane Centre, NHS R&D Programme, Summertown Pavillion, Oxford OX2 7LG, UK

Leslie E. Hughes
Department of Surgery, University of Wales College of Medicine, Heath Park, Cardiff CF4 4XN, UK

Knud Kragballe
Department of Dermatology, Marselisborg Hospital, 8000 Aarhus C, Denmark

Sean W. Lanigan
Department of Dermatology, Bridgend General Hospital, Quarella Road, Bridgend, Mid Glamorgan CF31 1JP, UK

Clifford Lawrence
Department of Dermatology, Royal Victoria Infirmary, Newcastle upon Tyne NE1 4LP, UK

Nicholas J. Lowe
Skin Research Foundation of California, 2001 Santa Monica Boulevard, Santa Monica, California 90404 and UCLA School of Medicine, Los Angeles, California, USA

Thomas A. Luger
Department of Dermatology and Ludwig Boltzmann Institute for Cell Biology and Immunobiology of the Skin, University of Münster, 4400 Münster, Germany

Stephen H. Mandy
Department of Dermatology, University
of Miami, Florida; Aspen Skin Clinic,
430 W. Main, Aspen, Colorado 81611,
USA

Ronald Marks
Department of Dermatology, University
of Wales College of Medicine, Heath
Park, Cardiff CF4 4XN, UK

Richard J. Motley
Department of Dermatology, University
of Wales College of Medicine, Heath
Park, Cardiff CF4 4XN, UK

Louise Poskitt
Department of Dermatology, Amersham
General Hospital, Amersham HP7 0JD,
UK

Alan Rosenbach
Skin Research Foundation of California,
2001 Santa Monica Boulevard, Santa
Monica, California 90404, USA

Karen Simpson
Skin Research Foundation of California,
2001 Santa Monica Boulevard, Santa
Monica, California 90404, USA

Stephen E. Smith
Department of Clinical Pharmacology, St
Thomas's Hospital, London SE1 7EH,
UK

Fenella Wojnarowska
Department of Dermatology, The
Churchill Hospital, Oxford OX3 7LJ, UK

Introduction

Ronald Marks

It has to be admitted that dermatologists traditionally have been better known for their keen clinical diagnostic skills and their knowledge of the classification of skin disorder than for their ability to treat skin diseases effectively. We sincerely trust that because in the 1990s there are many more potent drugs available, as well as an improved appreciation of the pharmacology of many of the disease processes involved, the era of therapeutic impotence is at an end. We trust that this volume adds impetus to the trend toward rational treatments for patients with skin disease: it contains a series of individually complete essays on cutting-edge subjects, all of which are important to the management of patients with common dermatoses. Old 'tried and true' treatments are not ignored, and there are descriptions of the usefulness for skin disorders of some drugs not generally thought 'dermatological'. For the 'research-minded', there are the results of many recent studies and descriptions of the clinical-trial methodologies used.

New molecules for old diseases

Cyclosporin in the treatment of psoriasis

Lionel Fry

Introduction

Psoriasis has been shown to be a disorder of abnormal keratinocyte proliferation mediated by activated CD4 lymphocytes.[1] Thus cyclosporin (CyA) which has a selective action on activated CD4 cells inhibiting cytokine production, should prove an effective treatment in psoriasis. An early study[2] done over a period of 3 months did indeed show CyA to be an effective drug in clearing psoriasis. However, severe psoriasis tends to be a chronic disease, and like other treatments cyclosporin suppresses the disorder but does not alter the activity and natural history of the disease. Thus treatment in most patients has to be indefinite. Cyclosporin unfortunately is not without side-effects, the two most important being nephrotoxicity and hypertension. At St Mary's Hospital, Paddington, we have used cyclosporin in the treatment of psoriasis since 1985, and now report our experiences with this drug.

Method

Patients

Over the last 6.5 years we have treated 84 patients with psoriasis with CyA. The mean age of the patients was 43 years (range 18–76 years), there were 48 men and 36 women. Of these patients, 31 were treated with short courses (i.e. up to 3 months) of CyA; these patients are referred to here as the 'short-term group'. A total of 35 patients were treated long term i.e. for more than 1 year. These patients were divided into 2 groups: group I consisted of 25 patients treated for more than 1 year but less than 4 years (mean 2.1 years); and group II comprised 10 patients treated for 5.0–6.5 years (mean 6.0 years). The remaining 18 patients were treated for more than 3 months but less than 1 year.

Dose

The initial dose was 3 mg/kg per day, in the majority of patients. In very severe psoriasis the initial dose was 4 mg/kg per day. The dose was adjusted at each visit according to the clinical state of the disease. The aim was not total clearance, but to achieve a degree of clearance acceptable to the patient. The dose ranged from 1 to 6 mg/kg

per day. Only two patients received 6 mg/kg per day for short periods.

Clinical assessment

This was done by using the psoriasis area severity index (PASI) score.[3] The PASI was determined at each visit.

Frequency of visits

At the beginning of treatment patients were seen every 2 weeks for the first 2 months and then monthly for the next 4 months. Once the long-term patients had been established on a maintenance dose, they were seen every 6 weeks, unless complications occurred, in which case they were seen more frequently.

Monitoring

Prior to treatment a detailed medical history was taken. Blood pressure was recorded at each visit. A full blood count, liver function tests, serum creatinine, and urine analysis were performed prior to treatment, and (except for the full blood count) at each subsequent visit. During the first 2 years of using CyA, no other test of renal function was performed. However, during the last 4.5 years glomerular filtration (GFR) was estimated prior to the initiation of treatment, and every 6 months subsequently. Renal biopsies were performed in eight patients after 5 years of treatment.

Results

Efficacy

The average reduction in the PASI for all patients was 69%. The maintenance dose, for satisfactory control of the psoriasis, was 1–2 in 15%, 3 in 40%, 4 in 25%, and 5 mg/kg per day in 14%. Five patients (6%) could not be controlled with a maintenance dose of 5 mg/kg per day, and treatment was discontinued. In these five patients, the psoriasis did clear with a higher dose, which showed that the disease was still responsive to CyA. However, side-effects are related to the dose and it was considered unwise to continue with CyA. The average maintenance dose for all patients was 3.3 mg/kg per day. The dose required to achieve satisfactory clearance fluctuates over a period of time and thus the dose should always be reduced if the disease is minimal. Conversely, if the psoriasis should become more severe the dose can be increased to 5 mg/kg per day. It is unwise to exceed this dose for any length of time.

Adjuvant therapy

Topical treatment with steroids, dithranol and calcipotriol was used, if patients had small areas of resistant psoriasis and it was thought unwise to increase the dose of CyA. In two patients etretinate was given in addition to CyA, but this did not have any additional benefit. Etretinate was used for only up to 3 months. It was considered unwise to combine CyA with methotrexate, as CyA is metabolized in the liver and is nephrotoxic, and methotrexate is hepatotoxic and is excreted by the kidneys. Ultraviolet radiation (PUVA and UVB) were not used as adjuvant therapy as both are potentially carcinogenic and, as CyA is an immunosuppressive agent, their combined use could theoretically increase the risk of the development of skin malignancies.

Discontinuation of treatment

CyA treatment had to be stopped in 13 patients (14%). In five patients there was significant impairment of renal function; in four there was poor compliance; two required a high dose of non-steroidal anti-inflammatory drugs (NSAIDs) to treat associated arthropathy (NSAIDs potentiate the nephrotoxicity of CyA) — in one because of severe nausea; and one patient (the eldest) died of a cerebrovascular accident after 3.5 years of treatment aged 79 years.

Side-effects

Minor side-effects included hirsutes, tremor, paraesthesiae, headache and lethargy. In none of the patients were these side-effects severe, so treatment was continued. Apart from the hirsutes, none of the side-effects were persistent.

Malignancy

Three of the 84 patients developed malignancies. One patient developed carcinoma *in situ* of the cervix after 2 years of treatment with CyA. The patient was treated with laser surgery, and has continued with CyA for another 4 years, and is still receiving treatment. Regular cervical smears have not shown any evidence of recurrence.

The second patient developed a squamous cell carcinoma and two basal cell carcinomas, all of which were treated surgically. CyA treatment was not discontinued.

The third patient developed two squamous cell carcinomas of the skin (she had a similar carcinoma prior to starting CyA). The lesions were treated surgically and treatment with CyA has not been discontinued.

The latter two patients had both received prolonged courses of UVB and PUVA, and one had received 10 years of treatment with methotrexate. Thus, what part CyA and what part the other treatments played in the development of the malignancies cannot be determined.

Hypertension

A total of 27 (32%) of the 84 patients developed hypertension (i.e. blood pressure >160/95). Two patterns of hypertension emerged. In the first the hypertension had an early onset, i.e. within the first 3 months of treatment. This occurred in 12 of the 27 patients. In the second pattern the blood pressure rose late in the treatment (from 1 to 4 years) and this occurred in 15 of the 27 patients. Initially, the dose of CyA was reduced in an attempt to lower the blood pressure, but if this was not possible hypotensive treatment was given. Nifedipine was the first drug of choice, as unlike other calcium channel blockers it does not interfere with the liver metabolism of CyA. In patients who developed side-effects to nifedipine or in whom it was not effective, beta blockers were used. None of the patients had to discontinue CyA because of hypertension. In all 27 patients the hypertension was reversed within 1 month of stopping CyA.

Nephrotoxicity

Serum creatinine

When monitoring renal function by serum creatinine, a *persistent* rise of more than 30% of the baseline value is taken to imply significant nephrotoxicity. Thus the baseline value is of paramount importance, and serum creatinine should be determined on at least two occasions before commencing CyA treatment. For all patients the mean rise in serum creatinine over a mean period of 18 months was 14.8%.

There was a correlation between the rise in creatinine and the duration of treatment ($r=0.49$, $p<0.05$).

During short courses of CyA (i.e. <3 months) none of the patients had a rise in creatinine of >30%. In group I (of the long-term treatment), two patients had a persistent rise of >30%; however, this fell to below the 30% level when CyA was discontinued for 1 month. In group II, two of the 10 patients had a rise of creatinine of >30% and another two had a rise of >50%. When CyA was discontinued for 1 month, creatinine fell below the 30% level in the former two patients, but in the latter two creatinine decreased below 50% but was still above 30% of the baseline value.

Glomerular filtration rate

There was a fall in the GFR during treatment, the decrease correlating with the duration of treatment ($r=0.41$, $p<0.05$). In group I of the long-term patients, the GFR decreased by >10% in 75% of patients, by >20% in 60%, by >30% in 30%, and by 50% in 5%. When CyA was discontinued for 1 month, the GFR rose in all patients. However, a decrease of >20% of the baseline value was still present in 45% in patients, although no patient had a decrease of >30%. Thus, although the GFR level improved when CyA was discontinued for 1 month, the value did not return to the pretreatment level in all patients.

Renal biopsies

The features associated with CyA nephrotoxicity are increased interstitial fibrosis, hyaline deposits in the walls of the arterioles, tubular atrophy, and increased glomerular obsolescence. Of the eight patients who had renal biopsies after 5 years of treatment, two showed all four features, two showed three, two showed two, and two showed no abnormality. Only in the two patients showing all four features were the features considered to be of moderate severity, which warranted discontinuing CyA treatment. In the four patients showing some features of CyA nephrotoxicity, the changes were considered minimal, and CyA treatment was continued.

Correlation between biopsy findings and renal function

There was a good correlation between the biopsy findings and renal function studies. The two patients showing the largest renal biopsy changes both had a low GFR for their age, which failed to show a significant improvement when CyA was discontinued for 1 month. In addition, both showed a rise in serum creatinine of >30%. Thus renal biopsies are not necessary in the routine management of patients receiving long-term CyA treatment for psoriasis. It should be possible to monitor patients by measuring serum creatinine and GFR. In patients who show a persistent rise in creatinine of

>30%, and those who show a fall in GFR of >40%, CyA should be discontinued until the creatinine level and GFR return to their pretreatment values.

Follow-up patients with impaired renal function

In the five patients in whom CyA treatment had to be discontinued because of impairment of renal function, follow-up tests were performed 6 months after discontinuing treatment. Four of the five patients had a >30% rise in creatinine when treatment was stopped, but in only one patient this rise was maintained after 6 months. After 6 months the GFR had fallen by >35% in all five patients. After 6 months of stopping CyA, the GFR improved in all patients, but still showed a fall of >35% in one, and of >25% in three patients. In only one patient had it returned to the pretreatment value. Thus, although renal function improved when CyA was discontinued for 6 months, the pretreatment values of creatinine and GFR were only achieved in one patient.

should not exceed 5 mg/kg per day. Patients not responding to this dose should discontinue CyA and receive alternative therapy.

Hypertension is a common complication and there are two patterns: in 15% of patients hypertension occurred within 3 months of commencing treatment; and in 17% of patients it occurred after a long period (i.e. >1 year) of CyA treatment.

Some impairment of renal function, as measured by GFR, occurred in the majority of patients after 2 years of treatment. This improved when CyA was discontinued for 1 month, but did not return to the pretreatment value in all patients.

Renal biopsy showed moderate features of CyA nephrotoxicity in two of eight patients after 5 years of CyA treatment. There was good correlation between renal biopsy findings and tests of renal function.

In patients in whom CyA treatment was discontinued because of nephrotoxicity and who were followed-up for 6 months, improvement in renal function occurred. However, in only one of the five patients in this study who discontinued CyA did the function return to pretreatment levels.

Summary

CyA is an effective treatment for severe psoriasis. The initial dose should be 3 mg/kg per day, and should be altered according to the clinical state of the psoriasis. The average maintenance dose was 3.3 mg/kg per day. The dose

References

1 **Valdimarsson H, Baker BS, Jonsdottir I, Fry L,** Psoriasis: a disorder of abnormal keratinocyte proliferation induced by T lymphocytes, *Immunol Today* (1986) 7: 256–9.

2 Griffiths CEM, Powles AV, Leonard JN et al, Clearance of psoriasis with low dose cyclosporin, *Br Med J* (1986) **293**: 731–2.

3 Fredriksson T, Pettersson U, Severe psoriasis — oral therapy with a new retinoid, *Dermatologica* (1978) **157**: 238–44.

2

New antifungal agents

Roderick J. Hay

Abstract

While the past 10 years have seen a major expansion in the number of antifungal drugs, there are still areas for improvement in both the range and scope of antifungal chemotherapy. New developments in this field have included the modification of existing drug molecules in order to eliminate toxicity and improve the spectrum of activity, for instance with the development of the triazoles from the imidazoles, or the use of less toxic formulations including the amphotericin B lipid complexes. The development of new groups of drugs with different modes of action such as the morpholines and the echinocandins has also been possible. In the superficial mycoses it has been possible to reduce the duration of therapy and to combat diseases such as onychomycosis where, previously, the success rate of treatment was low.

Introduction

The fungal infections or mycoses range from the commonplace (oral candidosis, tinea pedis) to rare systemic diseases such as systemic penicillinosis seen in some AIDS patients. When considering therapy, though, it is important to realize that, compared with the large number of antibacterial drugs, there are far fewer antifungals which belong to three main families (the polyenes, the azoles and the allylamines). There is also a miscellaneous group of compounds (including flucytosine and griseofulvin) which do not belong to a single family of drugs. This is not a static picture and there are new groups of antifungals under development all the time. These include the new azole or polyene derivatives, the morpholine antifungals such as amorolfine, a new fungal sterol biosynthesis inhibitor,[1] and cell wall antagonists such as the echinocandins (e.g. cilofungin[2]) and the nikkomycins.

Polyene antifungals

The polyene antifungals comprise a large family of drugs which are derived from *Streptomycete* species,[3] but only three (amphotericin B, nystatin and natamycin) are used in human disease. The activity of the polyene antifungals depends on the inhibition of the formation of the fungal cell membrane. Their lethal effect can be separated from an increase in cell permeability which is reversible at low concentrations.[3]

Similar binding to cholesterol in mammalian cell membranes is believed to form the basis of their toxicity in man. As topical therapies, the polyenes are principally used for superficial candidosis. They are less effective in established AIDS cases where orally absorbed drugs for oropharyngeal candidosis are necessary. The only drug of this series which can be given parenterally is amphotericin B. It disappears rapidly from serum and is thought to be bound thereafter to tissue cell membranes.[4] Amphotericin B has a broad range of antifungal activity, including the major pathogens involved in systemic mycoses, apart from the zygomycete fungi. Amphotericin B can be used topically or is given intravenously in 5% dextrose, but is commonly toxic.[5] The side-effects of amphotericin B include immediate reactions of hyperpyrexia, severe malaise and hypotension; acute renal failure, anaemia and hypokalaemia have also been recorded.[6]

Recent developments include the development of amphotericin B analogues, such as ester derivatives and reformulation of the drug in a different vehicle. An attempt has been made to avoid the side-effects of amphotericin B by incorporating the drug into liposomes[7,8] or lipid complexes. One less toxic unilamellar liposomal preparation of amphotericin B (Ambisome) is now available in some countries for seriously ill patients with systemic mycoses.[9] Other lipid formulations under investigation include a lipid complex (ABLC) and a colloidal dispersion (ABCD). These have little value in superficial mycoses and are costly.

The azole antifungals

The azole antifungals are a rapidly expanding family of drugs.[10] The first group to be developed, the imidazoles, contains a large number of compounds primarily aimed at topical use. The only members available for parenteral or systemic usage are miconazole, which can be administered intravenously, and ketoconazole which can be given orally. The principal mode of action of this series is the inhibition of cytochrome P450 dependent C14 demethylation in the formation of ergosterol in the fungal cell membrane. One of the potential disadvantages of this group is that in many cases there is some interference with human cytochrome P450 as well,[11] affecting some human metabolic processes. Ketoconazole, for instance, is a potent blocker of adrenal androgen biosynthesis and also effects prostacycline/leukotriene biosynthesis. The imidazoles vary considerably in their absorption after oral administration and the doses of both ketoconazole and itraconazole have to be increased in patients with AIDS and in bone marrow transplant recipients.

The newer triazole series (fluconazole, itraconazole and terconazole) act by the same mechanism as the imidazoles, i.e. via inhibition of cytochrome P450. The triazoles in current use are said to have less affinity at therapeutic levels with mammalian cytochrome P450, although there may be variation between individual triazoles in this respect. Adverse effects due to blockade of human cytochrome P450 have not been reported with these drugs.[11,12]

Fluconazole, being very water soluble, has excellent absorption and is widely distributed throughout the body.[12] Reduction in dosage is advised in patients with renal impairment. An intravenous preparation of this azole is also available. Although itraconazole is absorbed in low concentrations, tissue levels in liver, brain and skin[13] are considerably higher and there is evidence that in many of these sites there is prolonged elimination. The most dramatic example of this is the nails, where levels of drug can be detected 3 months after the end of therapy.

The imidazole antifungals affect most of the common superficial fungal pathogens. For superficial infection they are available as 1% creams, ointments or powders, although some special formulations are available, e.g. ketoconazole shampoo (seborrhoeic dermatitis) and econazole powder spray (tinea pedis). In addition, ketoconazole is active via the oral route in doses of 200–400 mg, but its use in long-term therapy, for instance for onychomycosis, is limited because of the risk of hepatoxicity estimated to occur in about 1:10 000 cases. It is, however, effective after a single dose in vaginal candidosis and pityriasis versicolor. An important feature of fluconazole is its speed of action. For instance, a single dose of 150 mg fluconazole rapidly induces clinical and mycological remission in over 90% of patients with vaginal candidosis.[14] Rapid responses are also seen with oral therapy (50 mg daily) for oropharyngeal candidosis (Fig. 2.1) in HIV infections.[15] Similar rapid responses of oral candidosis have been seen in neutropenic cancer patients. Remission in patients with chronic mucocutaneous candidosis has been seen to occur within 5 days.[16]

Itraconazole has been most fully assessed in the superficial mycoses[17] where it is effective in dermatophytosis, pityriasis versicolor and candidosis. The usual courses given in dermatophytosis (Fig. 2.2) are 14 days (100 mg daily) for tinea corporis or tinea cruris, and 30 days for tinea pedis. In pityriasis versicolor a dose of 800–1000 mg is necessary to produce a response; in vaginal candidosis 600 mg can be given over a single day as an effective therapy. Comparative studies indicate that itraconazole has some advantages over griseofulvin, particularly in tinea corporis, and preliminary data on nails show that it is useful where there has been no response to griseofulvin.[18] Given that the drug is retained in nails, it should be possible to use treatments of limited duration in onychomycosis; this has now been established using 3 months of therapy for onychomycosis of the toe-nails.[19] Itraconazole is also active in certain subcutaneous infections such as sporotrichosis and chromomycosis,[20] but it has little effect in mycetoma.

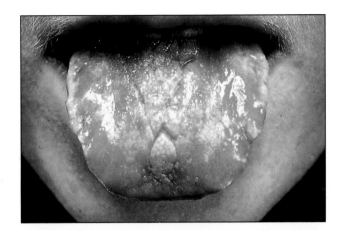

Figure 2.1
Chronic oral candidosis.

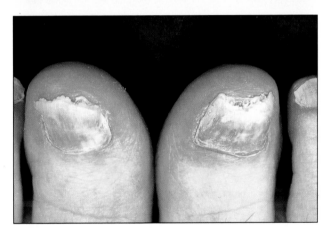

Figure 2.2
Dermatophytosis.

In systemic infections the uses of the azoles are less well established. Few are active, however, against aspergilli and zygomycetes, e.g. fluconazole. Itraconazole is active against a broader spectrum of fungi with the possible exception of the zygomycetes. Cryptococcal meningitis in AIDS patients responds to fluconazole both as initial and as suppressive therapy,[21] and the same drug is helpful in treating those with soft tissue cryptococcosis. As itraconazole penetrates the cerebrospinal fluid only very poorly, its use in cryptococcal meningitis has been questioned on theoretical grounds. However, in practice, at high dosage, and particularly if combined with flucytosine, it can induce remission.[22]

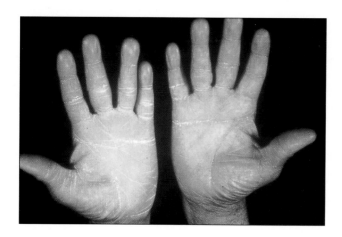

Figure 2.3

Trichophyton rubrum infection on the palms.

The final area of use for azoles (in this case mainly fluconazole) is in oral antifungal prophylaxis.[12] It has, however, been shown that other potentially pathogenic *Candida* species such as *C. krusei* may emerge, either in superficial or gastrointestinal carriage or causing true infections; *C. krusei* and *C. glabrata*, for instance are often less sensitive *in vitro* to the drug, suggesting that some form of selection has taken place. A new oral formulation of itraconazole in cyclodextrin has now been developed which is better absorbed in the neutropenic patient.

The allylamines

There are two allylamine antifungals in current use: naftifine and terbinafine.[23] The allylamines appear to have a similar site of action in the cell membrane as the tolcyclate antifungals, such as tolnaftate, squalene epoxidase. This step is, therefore, not affected by blockade or cytochrome P450. While naftifine has both antifungal and anti-inflammatory activity, the fungicidal concentrations (MFCs) of terbinafine are very similar to those required for mere inhibition of growth (MICs) *in vitro*. The main clinical use of terbinafine is in dermatophyte infections, but *in vitro* it has activity against *Aspergillus* and some of the dimorphic pathogens, such as *Histoplasma* and *Blastomyces*. Terbinafine is effective against dermatophytes when given orally and against a slightly broader range of superficial pathogens including *Pityrosporum* yeasts when applied topically. In one comparative study of terbinafine (250 mg twice daily) versus griseofulvin (500 mg twice daily) in chronic dry type tinea pedis caused by *Trichophyton rubrum* (Fig. 2.3), only

45% of the griseofulvin treated patients achieved remission 12 weeks after the end of therapy compared with 100% in the terbinafine group.[24] Other similar studies confirm this high recovery rate in infections of the skin. Onychomycosis also responds well to therapy with terbinafine,[25] with a very low relapse rate. The duration of therapy has now been established as 6 weeks for finger-nail and 12 weeks for toe-nail infections.[26] In both instances treatment is stopped before clinical recovery. The therapeutic range may be greater than this and, for instance, activity in *C. parapsilosis* paronychia and sporotrichosis have been recorded.

Other antifungal agents

There is a large and miscellaneous group of antifungal agents, many of which are only available for topical use. These include compounds such as tolnaftate, cyclopiroxolamine and haloprogin, all of which are effective treatments for superficial mycoses, although the activity of tolnaftate is confined to the dermatophytes. Griseofulvin, an oral agent which acts by the inhibition of intracellular microtubule formation, is widely used for dermatophytosis and is the treatment of choice for scalp infections. While in finger-nail infection griseofulvin produces over 70% remission rates, it has been less useful in toe-nail disease. For instance, one long-term study found a 30% remission rate in patients receiving up to 2 years of therapy.[27]

Flucytosine is still widely used in systemic antifungal chemotherapy. It interferes with the formation of RNA and DNA, but is actively taken up by fungi via a permease system and is converted to fluorouracil within the cell.

At present there are no clinical data on the value of the inhibitors of cell wall synthesis such as the echinocandins and nikkomycin derivatives.

Amorolfine, a new morpholine antifungal agent, is topically active against a variety of superficial pathogenic fungi from *Candida* to dermatophytes. It appears to block the production of cell membrane ergosterol via the inhibition of at least two separate steps: the 1,4 reductase and the 7,8 isomerase stages.[1] In a multi-centre study of 456 patients with onychomycosis, a 5% amorolfine nail lacquer given twice weekly for up to 6 months produced a clinical response rate of 54%, 3 months after the end of therapy. While the duration of follow-up was comparatively short, this study has produced encouraging results for the treatment of nail disease. Patients entering the study had early nail infections, not affecting more than 80% of the nail surface area and not involving the nail bed.[28]

Discussion

The current range of antifungal drugs, although extensive, is by no means ideal. There are, for instance, several mycoses which are refractory to existing

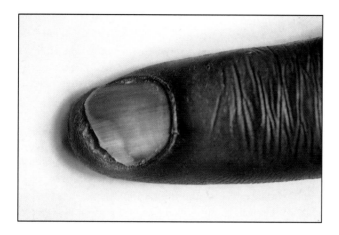

Figure 2.4

Hendersonula toruloidea infection of the nail.

therapy. Examples include common conditions such as chronic tinea pedis due to *Trichophyton rubrum*, and onychomycosis, although some of the newer additions such as short-term terbinafine and itraconazole administration may provide an answer. The topical approach to the treatment of nail disease has been more disappointing, despite evidence that by using penetration enhancers it is possible to obtain active concentrations *in vitro* at the site of fungal invasion; the new 5% nail lacquer of amorolfine has been reported to produce better responses. There are still some untreatable superficial mycoses such as those caused by *Scytalidium dimidiatum* (*Hendersonula toruloidea*, Fig. 2.4) and *S. hyalinum*.

Drug resistance to antifungal agents is rare,[29] apart from flucytosine where primary and secondary resistant yeasts are seen frequently in clinical practice. Polyene antifungal resistance is extremely rare but has been recorded. Azole resistance has been reported in patients receiving long-term ketoconazole therapy. It has been described mainly in patients with chronic mucocutaneous candidosis and in those with AIDS. While in some instances the 'resistance' cannot be substantiated, as it has not proved possible to compare pre- and post-therapy isolates, there is little doubt that resistance can appear in the chronic mucocutaneous candidosis group, at least. These resistant organisms may show cross-resistance to other azoles. Patients infected by yeasts in which this has occurred may still respond clinically to therapy with ketoconazole or other azoles, although not as well, and there is no evidence that the organism recovers its original sensitivity. Recently, fluconazole resistance has been reported in strains of *C. glabrata*[30] as well as other *Candida* species.

References

1 Polak A, Mode of action of the morpholine derivatives, *Ann NY Acad Sci* (1988) **544**: 221–8.

2 Debono M, Abbott BJ, Turner JR et al, Synthesis and evaluation of LY 121019, a member of a series of semisynthetic analogues of the antifungal lipopeptide, echinocandin B, *Ann NY Acad Sci* (1988) **544**: 141–7.

3 Medoff G, Kobayashi GA, The polyenes. In: Speller DCE (ed). *Antifungal chemotherapy*, Chichester: Wiley, 1980, pp. 3–34.

4 Bindschadler DD, Bennett JE, A pharmacological guide to the clinical use of amphotericin B, *J Infect Dis* (1961) **120**: 427–35.

5 Miller R, Bates JH, Amphotericin B toxicity. A follow up report of 53 patients, *Ann Intern Med* (1969) **71**: 1090–5.

6 Butler WT, Bennett JE, Alling D, Wertlake PT, Nephrotoxicity of amphotericin B: early and late effects in 81 patients, *Ann Intern Med* (1964) **61**: 175–87.

7 Lopez-Berestein G, Fainstein V, Hopfer R et al, Liposomal amphotericin B for the treatment of systemic fungal infections in patients with cancer: a preliminary study. *J Infect Dis* (1987) **151**: 704–10.

8 Sculier J-P, Coune A, Meunier F et al, Pilot study of amphotericin B entrapped in sonicated liposomes in cancer patients with fungal infections, *Eur J Cancer Clin Oncol* (1988) **24**: 527–38.

9 Hay RJ, Clinical assessment of liposomal amphotericin B, in *1st International Conference on Antifungal Chemotherapy, Tokyo, 1992*, Tokyo 1992, abs. 34.

10 Fromtling RA, Overview of medically important antifungal azole derivatives. *Clin Microbiol Rev* (1988) **1**: 187–217.

11 Grant SM, Clissold SP, Itraconazole: a review of its pharmacodynamic and pharmacokinetic properties and therapeutic use in superficial and systemic mycoses, *Drugs* (1989) **37**: 310–44.

12 Grant SM, Clissold SP, Fluconazole. A review of its pharmacodynamic and pharmacokinetic properties and therapeutic use in superficial and systemic mycoses, *Drugs* (1990) **39**: 877–901.

13 Heykants J, Van Peer A, Van de Velde V et al, The clinical pharmacokinetics of itraconazole: an overview, *Mycoses* (1989) **32** (Suppl. 1): 67–87.

14 Brammer KW, Lees LJ, Single dose oral fluconazole in the treatment of vulvovaginal candidiasis: an interim analysis of a comparative study versus three-day intravaginal clotrimazole tablets. In: Fromtling RA (ed). *Recent trends in the discovery, development and evaluation of antifungal agents.* Barcelona: JR Prous, 1987, pp. 151–6.

15 Dupont B, Drouhet E, Fluconazole in the management of oropharyngeal candidosis in a predominantly HIV antibody positive group of patients, *J Med Vet Mycol* (1988) **26**: 67–71.

16 Hay RJ, Clayton YM, Moore MK, Midgley G, Fluconazole in chronic mucocutaneous candidosis, *Br J Dermatol* (1988) **119**: 683–4.

17 Degreef H, Marien K, de Veylder H et al, Itraconazole in the treatment of dermatophytoses: an overview, *Rev Infect Dis* (1987) **9** (Suppl. 1): 104–8.

18 Hay RJ, Clayton YM, Moore MK, Midgley G, An evaluation of itraconazole in onychomycosis, *Br J Dermatol* (1988) 119: 359–66.

19 Willemsen M, de Doncker P, Willems J et al, Post treatment itraconazole levels in the nail: new implications for treatment, *J Am Acad Dermatol* (1992) 26: 731–5.

20 Restrepo A, Robledo J, Gomez I et al, Itraconazole therapy in lymphangitic and cutaneous sporotrichosis, *Arch Dermatol* (1986) 122: 413–17.

21 Bozzette SA, Larsen RA, Chiu J et al, A placebo-controlled trial of maintenance therapy with fluconazole after treatment of cryptococcal meningitis in the acquired immunodeficiency syndrome, *N Engl J Med* (1991) 324: 580–4.

22 Viviani MA, Tortorano AM, Langer M et al, Experience with itraconazole in cryptococcosis and aspergillosis, *J Infection* (1989) 18: 151–65.

23 Petranyi G, Meingassner JG, Mieth H, Antifungal activity of the allylamine derivative, terbinafine *in vitro*, *Antimicrob Agents Chemother* (1987) 31: 1365–8.

24 Hay RJ, Logan R, Clayton YM et al, A comparative study of terbinafine versus griseofulvin in dry-type dermatophyte infections, *J Am Acad Dermatol* (1991) 24: 243–6.

25 Goodfield MJD, Rowell NR, Forster RA et al, Treatment of dermatophyte infections of the finger of toe nails with terbinafine (SF 86-327, Lamisil) an orally active fungicidal agent, *Br J Dermatol* (1989) 121: 753–7.

26 Goodfield MJD, Short duration therapy with terbinafine for dermatophyte onychomycosis: a multi-centre study, *Br J Dermatol* (1992) 126 (Suppl. 39): 33–5.

27 Davies RR, Everall JD, Hamilton E, Mycological and clinical evaluation of griseofulvin for chronic onychomycosis, *Br Med J* (1967) iii: 464–8.

28 Reinel D, Topical treatment of onychomycosis with amorolfine 5% nail lacquer: comparative efficacy and tolerability of once and twice weekly use, *Dermatology* (1992) 182 (Suppl.): 21–6.

29 Kerridge D, Fasoli M, Wayman FJ, Drug resistance in *Candida albicans* and *Candida glabrata*, *Annl NY Acad Sci* (1988) 544: 245–59.

30 Warnock DW, Burke J, Cope NJ et al, Fluconazole resistance in *Candida glabrata*, *Lancet* (1988) ii: 1310.

3

Advances in photochemotherapy

Nicholas J. Lowe, Karen Simpson, Alan Rosenbach and Marcia Baum

Introduction

Psoralen photochemotherapy has been in use for a variety of dermatologic diseases since the early 1970s.[1] It is a highly effective therapy for many patients. Refinement and development of alternative psoralens, alternative delivery routes for psoralens, and different ultraviolet radiation (UV) sources have helped to refine this therapy. This chapter reviews areas of refinement of psoralen photochemotherapy in the treatment of psoriasis.

Effects of different UV radiation sources and wavelengths on PUVA efficacy

Previous studies[2] that showed the peak of the erythema spectrum for psoralen erythema to lie at 365 nm have more recently proved to be inaccurate. Most of the more recent research has shown the action wavelength of 8-methoxypsoralen (8-MOP) and trimetholpsoralen (TMP) to be 335 nm rather than 365 nm.[3] The most efficient wavelengths for clearing psoriasis have also most recently been shown to be 335 nm rather than 365 nm.[4]

Most of the UV radiation apparatus used for PUVA photochemotherapy have their peak output in the longer wavelength UVA range, peaking usually at 360–365 nm. These machines emit relatively smaller amounts of the shorter wavelength UVA. More recently, Farr has shown that UV lamps filtered to emit wavelengths at 325 nm rather than at longer UVA wavelengths resulted in a greater degree of clearance of psoriasis in patients being treated with oral 8-MOP photochemotherapy.[5]

We also have compared two different UV radiation wavelength ranges in terms of their antipsoriasis efficacy. In our studies, the UV apparatus used were metal halide units (Dermalight 2000-3, Studio City, CA). The apparatus was equipped with two different UV glass filters that allowed wavelengths of either 295–400 nm (UVAB) or 320–400 nm (UVA). These two different spectra allowed more UVB and lower wavelength UVA (PUVAB) to be compared with longer wavelength UVA (PUVA). Patients were randomly assigned to either UV radiation treatment groups. Patients were graded according to overall severity of psoriasis

Table 3.1 Comparison of PUVA and PUVAB radiation in combination with oral 8-MOP + metal halide comparison of (PUVA) with (PUVAB)

	PUVAB 295–400 nm (n = 15)	PUVA 320–400 nm (n = 15)
No. of patients achieving clearance or >75% improvement	10/15	7/15
>50% improvement	13/15	10/15
Mean no. of treatments	16	25

using a scale of 0 (no disease) to 3 (severe disease) for erythema and induration. The overall global severity was evaluated. Response to therapy was rated as 'clear' or 'excellent' if there was greater than 75% improvement in psoriasis severity, 'moderate' if there was 25–50% improvement, and 'poor' if there was less than 25% improvement.

The results are summarized in Table 3.1. More patients receiving PUVAB (which includes UVB and the shorter wavelength UVA) showed greater than 50% improvement or clearance compared with PUVA treated patients. These preliminary studies suggest that adding UVB and shorter wavelength UVA to PUVA results in more efficient phototherapy for psoriasis.

Alternative oral psoralens in oral photochemotherapy of psoriasis

The two major types of oral psoralen currently in clinical use in the photochemotherapy of psoriasis are 8-methoxypsoralen (8-MOP) and 5-methoxypsoralen (5-MOP). Both are synthetic compounds, with methoxy groups at the 8 and 5 positions, respectively. 8-MOP is available and widely used clinically in the USA and Europe. 8-MOP, however, shows problems in approximately 25% of individuals treated with this drug[6]—they develop nausea, mood changes, tiredness, depression, and malaise or flu-like syndromes. In some patients these symptoms are sufficiently severe to justify alternative therapy. In other patients where the symptoms are milder, an adjustment in the dose of 8-MOP or splitting of the dose may be sufficient to control the symptoms. If, despite such treatment changes, symptoms remain severe, the use of alternative psoralens such as 5-MOP has been proposed.

5-MOP has been shown[7] to be effective in psoriasis whilst being less likely to give the side-effects associated with oral 8-MOP photochemotherapy. The dose of 5-MOP given needs to be double that of 8-MOP. 8-MOP is given using a liquid filled capsule in the USA (Oxpsoralen Ultra), the dose usually being 0.5 mg/kg bodyweight given 1 to 1.25 h before UVA radiation. Less rapidly absorbed forms of 8-MOP require slightly larger dosages and longer times of ingestion prior to UVA phototherapy. 5-MOP dosing is based on a dose of 1.2 mg/kg body weight with ingestion 2 h prior to irradiation. The reasons for the need for higher doses of 5-MOP are unclear at this time, but may include a slower and less efficient gastrointestinal absorption of 5-MOP in its current oral delivery form.

Recent investigations[8] have shown that 5-MOP PUVA was highly effective in the treatment of moderate to severe psoriasis in a placebo vs. UVA controlled study involving 56 patients.

In addition, a study was performed on 20 patients intolerant to 8-MOP. In this study all patients given 5-MOP tolerated the drug. Whilst 95% of these patients had experienced severe nausea with 8-MOP, only 10% experienced mild nausea with 5-MOP. In addition, less than 10% of patients experienced fatigue, mood changes or unwanted pruritis with 5-MOP. Of the 26 patients tested, 24 responded to 5-MOP photochemotherapy (Lowe et al, unpublished observations).

These observations confirm the reports of the efficacy of 5-MOP PUVA. 5-MOP PUVA appears to be better tolerated than 8-MOP PUVA, but further research is required. 5-MOP PUVA is not at this time (January 1993) approved for use in the USA.

Bathwater delivery of psoralens

Bathwater delivery of 8-MOP and TMP has been used for several years in Scandinavia[9] and more recently in the USA.[6,10] Patients treated using bathwater psoralen respond well to therapy. There is no risk of systemic side-effects because of the minimal levels of absorption of the psoralen.[10] Bathwater delivered 8-MOP is less photoactive than bathwater delivered TMP. As a result, in patients treated either in the summer months or in a climate with high solar intensity (e.g. southern USA), it is probably advisable to use 8-MOP rather than TMP, thus lessening the risk of unwanted phototoxic reactions.

The concentrations of 8-MOP used and other details of therapy using bathwater delivery are given in Table 3.2. We have found this to be a reliable method of treatment where the patient either does not desire to take oral therapy or develops significant side-effects on oral 8-MOP. However, it is less convenient than oral PUVA photochemotherapy because of the requirement for bathing facilities in the treatment center and the time needed for bathwater immersion.

Table 3.2 Details of bathwater delivered psoralen therapy

Whole-body PUVA using 8-MOP

1. (*a*) 15 ml of 1% Oxpsoralen lotion or (*b*) 50 mg of Oxpsoralen Ultra capsules are dissolved in 50 cm³ of near-boiling water
2. Add above and disperse in 100 l of bathwater
3. Patient soaks in bath for (*a*) 15 or (*b*) 30 min
4. Patient dries and immediately begins UVA radiation treatment
5. Initial UVA treatment is based on minimum phototoxic dose or skin type

Local PUVA of hand and foot psoriasis using 8-MOP

1. 1 cm³ of Oxpsoralen 1% lotion
2. Add to 2 l of water in a bowl
3. Soak hands/feet for 30 min
4. Dry and immediately start UVA

Recent reports from multicenter Scandinavian studies suggest that TMP bathwater therapy carries a lower risk of cutaneous carcinoma compared with oral 8-MOP PUVA. Further long-term studies are required to confirm these observations.[11]

Summary

Photochemotherapy of psoriasis has now been available for about 20 years. It has proved to be a highly effective form of treatment that enables patients to lead active productive lives without the need for hospitalization. Concerns of long-term cutaneous toxicity have been confirmed with oral psoralen photochemotherapy and 8-MOP. These have included increased risk of squamous cell carcinoma, atypical lentigo and photoaged skin. There have been no reports of a higher risk of systemic toxicity.

References

1 Parrish JA, Fitzpatrick TB, Tanenbaum L et al, Photochemotherapy of psoriasis with oral methoxpsoralen and long wave ultraviolet light, *N Eng J Med* (1974) **291**: 1207–11.

2 Pathak MA, Kramer DM, Fitzpatrick TB, *Photobiology and photochemistry of furocoumaris in sunlight and man*, Tokyo: Tokyo University Press, pp. 335–68.

3 Cripps DJ, Lowe NJ, Lerner AB, Action spectra of topical psoralens. A re-evaluation, *Br J Dermatol* (1982) **107**: 77–82.

4 Brucke J, Taneu A, Ortel B et al, Relative efficacy of 335 and 365 nm radiation in photochemotherapy of psoriasis, *Br J Dermatol* (1991) **124**: 372–4.

5 Farr P, Efficiency of different UVA spectral in phototherapy of psoriasis. Presented at the International Congress of Dermatology, New York, June 1992.

6 Lowe NJ, May L, Weingarten DP, PUVA for psoriasis: comparison of oral and bathwater delivery of 8-MOP, *J Am Acad Dermatol* (1986) **14**: 754–60.

7   Tanew A, Ortel B, Rappersberger K, Honigsmann N, 5-Methoxypsoralen for photochemotherapy, *J Am Acad Dermatol* (1988) **18**: 333–8.

8   Rosenbach A, Osterkamp G, Lowe NJ, 5-Methoxysporalen plus UVA versus placebo plus UVA less psoralens, *Eurotext for psoriasis 1992*, New York: J. Libbey, 1992, p. 57 (Abstr.).

9   Fisher T, Alsins J, Treatment of psoriasis with trioxalen baths and dyspro-sium lamps, *Acta Derm Venereol (Stockh)* (1976) **56**: 383–90.

10   David M, Lowe NJ, Borok M, Halder R, 8-Methoxysporalen blood levels following bath-water delivered 8-MOP, *J Am Acad Dermatol* (1990) **23**: 931–2.

11   Lindeloff B, Sigurgeisson B, Tegner E et al, Comparison of the carcinogenic potential of trioxalen bath PUVA and oral methoxsalen PUVA, *Arch Dermatol* (1992) **10**: 1341–5.

4

Vitamin D_3 and its analogues— therapeutic use in skin disease

Knud Kragballe

Introduction

Mechanism of action

Vitamin D_3 receptors

The hormonal form of vitamin D (1,25-dihydroxy vitamin D_3; 1,25-$(OH)_2D_3$) assists in maintaining calcium homeostasis by mediating intestinal calcium absorption and bone calcium mobilization. The classical effects of vitamin D are mediated through a receptor coupled process.[1] Recently, a receptor for vitamin D has been demonstrated in a variety of tissues not previously regarded as targets for vitamin D. This has offered new approaches to the treatment of diseases previously not believed to be related to the vitamin. Prime examples are haematopoietic tissue, the skin and cancer of various origins. Vitamin D_3 is obtained in the diet or produced in the skin from 7-dehydrocholesterol on exposure to sunlight. Vitamin D_3 becomes biologically active after successive hydroxylations in the liver and in the kidney to 1,25-$(OH)_2D_3$. Substantial evidence suggests that 1,25-$(OH)_2D_3$ acts via an intracellular receptor protein. This vitamin D receptor is a member of the steroid, oestrogen and retinoid receptor gene family of proteins which mediate the transcriptional activities of the corresponding ligands. The vitamin D–receptor complex binds in the nucleus to the vitamin D responsive element on the gene. This binding requires a nuclear accessory factor and results either in the synthesis of specific RNA encoding proteins or in a repression of gene transcription. The skin contains a specific receptor for 1,25-$(OH)_2D_3$. Immunohistochemical studies of normal skin have shown vitamin D receptor antigens to be expressed in keratinocytes of all epidermal layers (except those of the stratum corneum) and in cells of epidermal appendages.[2] Furthermore, a high proportion of Langerhans cells, monocytes and T-lymphocytes in normal skin express vitamin D receptors. Because the antibody applied against the vitamin D receptor can react with other proteins, the results obtained by immunohistochemistry need to be confirmed. Furthermore, the skin may be an alternative source of 1,25-$(OH)_2D_3$. Thus, cultured neonatal human keratinocytes can produce 1,25-$(OH)_2D_3$ from 25-$(OH)D_3$.

Effects on epidermal keratinocytes

The effects of 1,25-(OH)$_2$D$_3$ on epidermal keratinocyte proliferation and differentiation have been studied thoroughly. At physiological concentrations, 1,25-(OH)$_2$D$_3$ causes a decrease in the proliferation of and an increase in the morphological and biochemical differentiation of cultured keratinocytes. The mechanisms by which 1,25-(OH)$_2$D$_3$ causes inhibitory effects on keratinocyte proliferation are not understood, but may involve effects on epidermal growth factor receptor, transforming growth factor β$_1$ or c-myc. The rapid increase in intracellular calcium levels induced by 1,25-(OH)$_2$D$_3$ may be important for its effect on keratinocyte differentiation.[3] 1,25-(OH)$_2$D$_3$ is also recognized to have immunoregulatory properties.

Effect on mononuclear cells

Defined actions of the hormone on human peripheral blood mononuclear cells include the inhibition of mitogen/antigen-stimulated proliferation and the inhibition of immunoglobulin production.[4,5] There is experimental evidence to suggest that the specific target of 1,25-(OH)$_2$D$_3$ is the T-helper/inducer lymphocyte[6] and that a significant portion of the antiproliferative effect is mediated by interleukin-2 (IL-2).[7] 1,25-(OH)$_2$D$_3$ also influences the ability of monocytes to provide signals important in T-lymphocyte activation. Thus, 1,25-(OH)$_2$D$_3$ decreases monocyte HLA-DR expression, monocyte antigen presentation[8] and monocyte promotion of T-cell proliferation.[9] These in vitro findings clearly illustrate that 1,25-(OH)$_2$D$_3$ has the potential to exert an immunosuppressive effect.

Other anti-inflammatory mechanisms

It is unclear whether 1,25-(OH)$_2$D$_3$ has an anti-inflammatory capacity. While 1,25-(OH)$_2$D$_3$ has no consistent effects on monocyte expression of adhesion molecules (LFA-1, LFA-3, ICAM-1 and CD 44) or production of the cytokines IL-1β or IL-6,[9] it inhibits IL-1 induced IL-8 production.[10] The inhibitory effect on IL-8 production includes that in cultured human keratinocytes and fibroblasts.[10] The potential importance of these findings stems from the fact that IL-8 is present in inflammatory skin diseases such as psoriasis.

The effect of 1,25-(OH)$_2$D$_3$ on the skin immune system has been studied in the human allogeneic mixed epidermal cell lymphocyte reaction (MECLR).[11] In this reaction 1,25-(OH)$_2$D$_3$ causes an inhibition, which is maximal at a concentration of 10^{-8} M. In experiments designed to assess the effects of 1,25-(OH)$_2$D$_3$ on the two cell populations involved in this reaction, 1,25-(OH)$_2$D$_3$ was found to affect preferentially the epidermal cells. In this in vitro model 1,25-(OH)$_2$D$_3$ may affect epidermal cell function by inhibiting keratinocyte expression of HLA-DR.[12] The potential relevance of these results is supported by studies of skin allograft survival. In mice treated systemically with 1α-(OH)D$_3$, a prodrug of $1,25$-(OH)D$_3$, skin allograft survival is significantly prolonged.

Treatment of psoriasis with vitamin D analogues

Oral 1α-hydroxy vitamin D$_3$ (1α-(OH)D$_3$)

It was a chance observation that stimulated interest in vitamin D$_3$ in psoriasis.[13] A patient received oral 1α-(OH)D$_3$ at a dose of 0.75 μg/day for osteoporosis. After 22 months the patient's psoriatic skin lesions were dramatically improved. Later the same group of investigators reported improvement in 13 out of 17 psoriatic patients treated with 1α-(OH)D$_3$ at a dose of 1 μg/day for 6 months.[14] In another open study, 10 of 15 patients improved during treatment with 1α-(OH)D$_3$ at a dose of 1 μg/day for 4–6 months.[15]

Until controlled trials including larger numbers of patients have been conducted, it is impossible to make any conclusions about the efficacy and safety of 1α-(OH)D$_3$ in treating psoriasis. Because 1α-(OH)D$_3$ is a prodrug of $1,25$-(OH)$_2$D$_3$, it must be anticipated that the safety profile will be similar to that for oral $1,25$-(OH)$_2$D$_3$, which is described below.

Oral 1,25-(OH)$_2$D$_3$

The antipsoriatic effect of oral $1,25$-(OH)$_2$D$_3$ has been assessed in open studies without controls.[14,16,17] Approximately half of the treated patients have shown some degree of improvement. Unfortunately, the reported studies included few patients.[14,16,17] There is a safety problem with oral $1,25$-(OH)$_2$D$_3$, as hypercalciuria is usually observed when the dosage exceeds 0.75 μg/day.[17] Although administration of $1,25$-(OH)$_2$D$_3$ as a single dose at bedtime may reduce the incidence of hypercalciuria, some patients may still have to be withdrawn because of this side-effect.[17]

It must, therefore, be concluded that the therapeutic index of $1,25$-(OH)$_2$D$_3$ is low and that a safe and effective dose has still not been established.

Topical 1,25-(OH)$_2$D$_3$

Treatment of psoriasis with topical $1,25$-(OH)$_2$D$_3$ has produced mixed results. In the initial open studies, an improvement was reported after applying 0.5 μg/g or 3 μg/g.[14,17] However, in double-blind studies applying similar low doses, no benefit was found compared with placebo.[18,19] Later, a dose-finding study showed 25 μg/g and 50 μg/g to be more effective than 5 µg/g and 10 µg/g.[20] Although the use of different doses and different vehicles makes it difficult to make a direct comparison between the studies, it appears that doses of 3 µg/g or above are effective when formulated in a petrolatum based ointment.[21,22] However, it remains to be determined whether such a dose is safe. In one study, 1,25-(OH)$_2$D$_3$ was applied twice daily at a concentration of 15 µg/g without producing side-effects.[21] However, in a comparison between 3 µg/g and 15 µg/g, the higher concentration caused hypercalciuria when the treated skin area exceeded 600–1200 cm^2.[22] It can, therefore, be concluded that topical 1,25-(OH)$_2$D$_3$ is efficaceous in psoriasis, but that its calcitropic effect may limit its clinical use.

Topical calcipotriol

Calcipotriol is a synthetic vitamin D analogue with potent cell regulating properties, but a lower risk of inducing calcium related side-effects. It is a 1,24-(OH)$_2$D$_3$ analogue containing a double bond and a ring structure in the side-chain. As a consequence of this modification of the side-chain, it is rapidly transformed into inactive metabolites. Because of these pharmacokinetic properties, calcipotriol is about 200 times less potent than 1,25-(OH)$_2$D$_3$ in producing hypercalcaemia and hypercalciuria after oral and intraperitoneal administration in rats. In contrast, calcipotriol and 1,25-(OH)$_2$D$_3$ are equipotent in their affin-

ity for the vitamin D receptor and in their *in vitro* effects.[3]

In double-blind, placebo-controlled studies, topical calcipotriol has been shown to improve psoriasis.[23–26] Maximum improvement was observed at a concentration of 50 µg/g.[25] When applied twice daily, the improvement is detectable within 1–2 weeks and maximal at 6–8 weeks. Most patients experience a marked improvement, although complete resolution of symptoms is seldomly seen (Figs 4.1, 4.2). In large multicentre studies conducted in several European countries and in Canada, calcipotriol ointment has been shown to be slightly more efficaceous than 0.1% β-methasone 17-valerate ointment[27,28] and short-contact dithranol treatment.[29]

Side-effect profile of Vitamin D analogues

The potential effect on systemic calcium metabolism is the principal dose-limiting factor in the use of vitamin D analogues. In studies with calcipotriol, patients were provided with a maximum of 100 g ointment per week. Used according to these guidelines, no change was detected in serum calcium levels. However, two cases of hypercalcaemia developed after the application of 400 g ointment over 10 days[28] and of 200 g ointment over 7 days.[30] Although a few days after stopping treatment the serum calcium normalized in both cases, these reports illustrate that the excessive use of

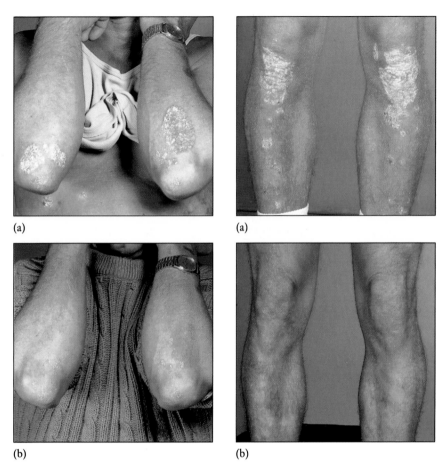

Figure 4.1

Photographs of a patient (a) before and (b) after treatment with topical calcipotriol. The patient shows a marked improvement.

Figure 4.2

Photographs of a patient (a) before and (b) after treatment with topical calcipotriol. The patient shows complete clearance.

calcipotriol may affect calcium metabolism.

Therefore, bone and calcium metabolism were studied in patients using calcipotriol according to the guidelines, i.e. less than 100 g per week. In a placebo-controlled study, patients treated with calcipotriol did not show a change in any of the parameters of calcium/bone metabolism compared with placebo-treated patients.[31] These results demonstrate that patients with psoriasis can be safely treated with topical calcipotriol. Skin irritation is seen in about 10% of patients treated with calcipotriol ointment. In most cases irritation is mild and may disappear during continued treatment. The face is particularly sensitive to calcipotriol ointment. Therefore, calcipotriol should, in general, not be used on the face.

Long-term use of calcipotriol

There is a gradual recurrence of psoriasis on stopping vitamin D treatment. Therefore, many patients require maintenance therapy. The long-term efficacy and safety of calcipotriol has been assessed in patients treated for 6–12 months. In a single-centre study, on average it was possible to maintain the induced improvement. The severity and incidence of side-effects were similar to those seen in short-term studies and neither hypercalcaemia nor skin atrophy developed.[28] Similar findings were made in a multicentre study (unpublished).

Combined therapies

Topical calcipotriol has also been evaluated in combination therapy of psoriasis. So far, calcipotriol treatment has been combined with UVB, PUVA and cyclosporin A. UVB phototherapy together with calcipotriol is more efficaceous than calcipotriol alone; in particular more patients experience a complete clearance of their disease.[33] Combination of calcipotriol with ultraviolet radiation (PUVA) increases the antipsoriatic effect (unpublished). Furthermore, low-dose cyclosporin A (2 mg/kg per day) given together with calcipotriol is more efficaceous than cyclosporin A alone (unpublished). The results of these trials suggest that addition of topical calcipotriol to UVB, PUVA and cyclosporin A not only improves the therapeutic efficacy, but also decreases the cumulative dose of ultraviolet light and cyclosporin A.

Topical 1,24-(OH)₂D₃

$1,24\text{-}(OH)_2D_3$ is another synthetic vitamin D₃ analogue developed for topical use in psoriasis. $1,24\text{-}(OH)_2D_3$ is equipotent with $1,25\text{-}(OH)_2D_3$ in its affinity for the vitamin D receptor and in its *in vitro* effects. Compared with $1,25\text{-}(OH)_2D_3$, less hypercalcaemia is induced after a single intravenous dose of $1,24\text{-}(OH)_2D_3$ in rats. However, the doses of $1,24\text{-}(OH)_2D_3$ and $1,25\text{-}(OH)_2D_3$ inducing hypercalcaemia are similar. These results indicate that $1,24\text{-}(OH)_2D_3$ may be advantageous over $1,25\text{-}(OH)_2D_3$, although less selective than calcipotriol.

Clinical experience with $1,24\text{-}(OH)_2D_3$ is rather limited. In an open study, $1,24\text{-}(OH)_2D_3$ ointment at doses of 1, 2 and 4 µg/g was applied under occlusion once daily. Within 1 month, $1,24\text{-}(OH)_2D_3$ produced improvement, irrespective of the concentration used.[34] The degree of improvement was similar to that observed with 0.1% β-methasone 17-valerate ointment. In a randomized, double-blind trial, $1,24\text{-}(OH)_2D_3$ containing either 1, 2 or 4 µg/g was applied to one side and 0.1% hydrocortisone butyrate or 0.1% β-methasone 17-valerate ointment to the contralateral side for 4 weeks. At the end of treatment, all three $1,24\text{-}(OH)_2D_3$ concentrations had produced a moderate or better improvement in about half of the patients.[35] There were no clinical side-effects or changes in serum calcium levels.

It appears that topical $1,24\text{-}(OH)_2D_3$ is effective for the short-term treatment of psoriasis. Because in the reported studies $1,24\text{-}(OH)_2D_3$ was only applied to limited skin areas, its safety profile remains to be determined.

Conclusions

Pharmacological doses of vitamin D_3 analogues have therapeutic effects in psoriasis. This application of vitamin D_3 is different from the classical use of vitamin D_3 as substitution therapy. Although there are conflicting results regarding vitamin D_3 metabolism in psoriasis, the present experimental data do not support the idea that psoriasis may be a manifestation of abnormal vitamin D_3 metabolism, either locally in the skin or systemically.

The mode of action of vitamin D analogues in psoriasis is not completely understood. The rationale for their use is their ability to reverse epidermal hyperproliferation and to promote epidermal differentiation. Because vitamin D analogues also possess immunosuppressive properties, it becomes important to assess whether their clinical effects may be partially attributed to their immune modulating properties. Another important question is whether it is possible to identify doses that are both efficacious and at the same time safe and well tolerated. With the availability of new vitamin D analogues with even more potent and selective activities, it may become possible to treat other hyperproliferative and immune mediated diseases of skin such as ichthyotic disorders, cancer, eczema and lupus erythematosus.

References

1 **Haussler MR**, Vitamin D receptors: nature and function, *Ann Rev Nutr* (1986) **6**: 527–62.

2 **Milde P, Hauser U, Simon T et al,** Expression of 1,25-dihydroxy-vitamin D_3 receptors in normal and psoriatic skin, *J Invest Dermatol* (1991) **97**: 230–6.

3 **Kragballe K**, Vitamin D_3 analogues in the treatment of psoriasis, *J Cell Biochem* (1992) **49**: 46–52.

4 **Tsoukas DD, Provvedini DM, Manolagas SC,** 1,25-Dihydroxyvitamin D_3: a novel immunoregulatory hormone, *Science* (1984) **224**: 1438–40.

5 Lemire JM, Adams JS, Sakai R, Jordan SC, 1,25-Dihydroxy-vitamin D$_3$ suppresses proliferation and immunoglobulin production by normal human peripheral blood mononuclear cells, *J Clin Invest* (1984) **74**: 657–61.

6 Lemire JM, Adams JS, Kermani-Arab V, 1,25-Dihydroxyvitamin D$_3$ suppresses human T helper/inducer lymphocyte activity *in vitro*, *J Immunol* (1985) **134**: 3032–5.

7 Rigby WFC, Stacy R, Fanger MW, Inhibition of T lymphocyte mitogenesis by 1,25-dihydroxyvitamin D$_3$ (calcitriol), *J Clin Invest* (1984) **74**: 1451–5.

8 Rigby WFC, Waugh MG, Graziano RF, Regulation of human monocyte HLA-DR and CD4 antigen expression and antigen presentation by 1,25-dihydroxyvitamin D$_3$, *Blood* (1990) **76**: 189–97.

9 Rigby WFC, Waugh MG, Decreased accessory cell function and costimulatory activity by 1,25-dihydroxyvitamin D$_3$-treated monocytes, *Arthritis Rheum* (1992) **35**: 110–9.

10 Larsen CG, Kristensen M, Paludan et al, 1,25-(OH)$_2$-D$_3$ regulator of interleukin-8 expression and production, *Biochem Biophys Res Commun* (1991) **176**: 1020–6.

11 Bagot M, Charue D, Pamphile R, Revux J, Immunosuppressive effects of 1,25-dihydroxyvitamin D$_3$ analogue (calcipotriol) on epidermal cells. In: Norman AW, Bouillon R, Thomasset M (eds). *Vitamin D: gene regulation structure–function analysis and clinical application.* Berlin: Walter de Gruyter, 1991, pp. 518–19.

12 Tani M, Komura A, Horkawa T, 1,25-Dihydroxyvitamin D$_3$ modulates Ia antigen expression induced by interferon-gamma and prostaglandin E$_2$ production in PAM 212 cells, *Br J Dermatol* (1992) **126**: 266–74.

13 Morimoto S, Yoshikawa K, A patient with psoriasis cured by 1-alpha-hydroxyvitamin D$_3$, *Med J Osaka Univ* (1985) **35**: 51–4.

14 Morimoto S, Yoshikawa K, Kozuka T et al, An open study of vitamin D$_3$ treatment in psoriasis vulgaris, *Br J Dermatol* (1986) **176**: 1020–6.

15 Holland DB, Wood EJ, Roberts SG et al, Epidermal cytokeratin levels during oral 1-alpha-hydroxyvitamin D$_3$ treatment for psoriasis, *Skin Pharmacol* (1989) **2**: 68–76.

16 Lugo-Somolinos A, Sanxhez JL, Haddock L, Efficacy of 1,25-dihydroxyvitamin D$_3$ (calcitriol) in the treatment of psoriasis vulgaris: an open study, *Bol Assoc Med PR* (1990) **82**: 450–3.

17 Smith EL, Pincus SH, Donovan L, Holick MF, A novel approach for the evaluation and treatment of psoriasis, *J Am Acad Dermatol* (1988) **19**: 360–4.

18 van de Kerkhof PCM, van Bokhoven M, Zultak M, Czarnetzki MB, A double-blind study of topical 1,25-dihydroxyvitamin D$_3$ in psoriasis, *Br J Dermatol* (1989) **120**: 661–4.

19 Henderson CA, Papworth-Smith J, Cunliffe WJ et al, A double-blind placebo-controlled trial of topical 1,25-dihydroxycalciferol in psoriasis, *Br J Dermatol* (1989) **121**: 493–6.

20 Ashenfelter A, Coutinho J, Gwo J et al, Calcitriol cream in the treatment of psoriasis: efficacy and safety considerations. In: *Proc. 4th International Psoriasis Symposium*, San Francisco, USA, 10–14 July, 1992, Abstract p. 108.

21 Holick MF, Pochi P, Bhawan J, Topically applied and orally administered 1,25-dihydroxyvitamin D_3 is a novel, safe, effective therapy for the treatment of psoriasis: a three year experience and histologic analysis, *J Invest Dermatol* (1989) **92**:446.

22 Langner A, Verjans H, Stapor V et al, Treatment of chronic plaque psoriasis by 1-alpha,25-dihydroxyvitamin D_3 ointment. In: Norman AW, Buillon R, Thomasset M (eds). *Vitamin D: gene regulation structure–function analysis and clinical application.* Berlin: Walter de Gruyter, 1991, pp. 430–1.

23 Kragballe K, Beck H-I, Søgaard H, Improvement of psoriasis by a topical vitamin D_3 analogue (MC 903) in a double-blind study, *Br J Dermatol* (1988) **199**: 223–30.

24 Staberg B, Roed-Pedersen J, Menne T, Efficacy of topical treatment in psoriasis with MC 903, a new vitamin D analogue, *Acta Derm Venereol (Stockh)* (1989) **69**: 147–50.

25 Kragballe K, Treatment of psoriasis by the topical application of the novel cholecalciferol analogue calcipotriol (MC 903), *Arch Dermatol* (1989) **125**: 1647–52.

26 Dubertret L, Wallach D, Souteyrand P et al, Efficacy and safety of calcipotriol (MC 903) ointment in psoriasis vulgaris, *J Am Acad Dermatol* (1992) **27**: 983–8.

27 Kragballe K, Gjertsen BT, De Hoope D et al, Double-blind, right-left comparison of calcipotriol and betamethasone valerate in treatment of psoriasis vulgaris, *Lancet* (1991) **337**: 193–6.

28 Cunliffe WJ, Claudy A, Fairiss G et al, A multicentre comparative study of calcipotriol and betamethasone 17-valerate in patients with psoriasis vulgaris, *J Am Acad Dermatol* (1992) **26**: 736–43.

29 Berth-Jones J, Chu AC, Dodd WAH et al, A multicentre parallel-group comparison of calcipotriol ointment and short-contact dithranol therapy in chronic plaque psoriasis, *Br J Dermatol* (1992) **127**: 266–71.

30 Dwyer C, Chapman RS, Calcipotriol and hypercalcemia, *Lancet* (1991) **338**: 764–5.

31 Mortensen L, Kragballe K, Schifter S, Charles P, Effect of calcipotriol on psoriasis: a double-blind, placebo-controlled study of calcipotriol (MC 903) and calcium metabolism. In: Norman AW, Buillon R, Thomasset M (eds). *Vitamin D: gene regulation structure–function analysis and clinical application.* Berlin: Walter de Gruyter, 1991, pp. 443–4.

32 Kragballe K, Fogh K, Long-term efficacy and tolerability of topical calcipotriol in psoriasis, *Acta Derm Venereol (Stockh)* (1991) **71**: 475–8.

33 Kragballe K, Combination of topical calcipotriol (MC 903) and UVB radiation for psoriasis, *Dermatologica* (1990) **181**: 211–4.

34 Kato T, Rokugo M, Terui T, Tagami H, Successful treatment of psoriasis with topical application of the active vitamin D_3 analogue, 1,24-dihydroxycholecalciferol, *Br J Dermatol* (1986) **115**: 431–3.

35 Tagami H, Kato T, Terui T, Tadaki T, Successful treatment of psoriasis with topical application of the active vitamin D_3 analog, 1 alpha,24-dihydroxycholecalciferol. In: Norman WA, Schaeffer K, Grigoleit H-G, Herrath D (eds). *Proc. Seventh Workshop on Vitamin D.* Berlin: Walter de Gruyter, 1988, pp. 958–67.

5

Cytokines—therapy of skin diseases

Thomas A. Luger

Introduction

Cytokines are a group of mediators which are rapidly and transiently produced upon activation by almost any cell. These secretory products play a crucial role during inflammation, immunological reactions, cell differentiation and tumour growth.[1] Therefore and with the present-day availability of recombinant molecules, cytokines recently have been introduced in the treatment of various skin diseases.

Interferons

Interferons in viral diseases

Based on their antiviral effects, interferons (IFN) have been widely used to treat viral diseases. In patients with frequent recurrences of herpes simplex virus infection, different schedules of subcutaneous and topical administration of recombinant IFNα have resulted in the suppression and/or decreased duration of the infection.[2] However, when the efficacy of IFNα for the treatment of first episode herpes genitalis was compared with topical acyclovir, it proved not to be superior in reducing the frequency or severity of relapses.[3] Placebo-controlled studies have shown a beneficial effect of IFNα and IFNβ on the clinical course of herpes zoster virus in immunocompromised patients.[2,4] When compared with acyclovir, IFNα turned out to be equally effective in herpes zoster virus. Side-effects, however, were observed more frequently in IFN treated patients than in those given acyclovir.[5]

Many studies have addressed the question of the efficacy of the effect of IFNs in the treatment of condylomata acuminata. Complete remission was observed in 30–50% of IFNα treated lesions versus a 15–30% response to placebo therapy.[2] Although monotherapy for condylomata acuminata with IFNα did not prove to be significantly superior to conventional therapy, adjuvant therapy with IFNα or IFNβ either topically or systemically after surgery, cryotherapy or laser treatment alone or in combination with retinoids appears to be promising.[2,6] Considering the published data, the beneficial effects of IFNγ in the treatment of condylomata acuminata are controversial.[2,7] With regard to bowenoid papulosis, preliminary data indicate that continuous treatment with IFNγ appears to be effective, showing a complete response in three of four patients.[8] Several studies have focused on IFN treatment for common warts, but its value is still uncertain. In contrast, epidermodysplasia verruciformis can be treated successfully with systemic IFNα; however, discontinuation of treatment results in rapid relapse.[2,9]

Interferons in cutaneous T-cell lymphomas

Recombinant IFNα, either alone or in combination with other therapeutic regimens, has been demonstrated to be effective in the treatment of cutaneous T-cell lymphomas. In initial studies, high dose IFNα (up to 5×10^7 U/m²) revealed a response rate of more than 50%.[10] In another randomized trial, low dose IFNα (3×10^6 U/m²) was compared with an increasing-dose regimen, resulting in an overall response of 68%.[11] Intralesional application of low dose IFNα into the plaques resulted in regression of most lesions, whereas systemic low dose IFNα (5×10^6 U three times weekly for 4 weeks) was not effective in five patients.[12] Promising data have recently been reported by several groups with the use of a combination of IFNα (18×10^6 U three times weekly) and retinoids (0.7 mg/kg per day) yielding a response rate of about 50%.[13–15] Concurrent treatment of IFNα (6–30 $\times 10^6$ U three times weekly) with ultraviolet radiation (PUVA) in 15 patients gave an overall response rate of 93%.[16] A beneficial effect of low dose IFNα and extracorporal photophoresis was recently observed in a patient with Sézary syndrome.[17] Combinations of IFNα with chemotherapeutic agents in the treatment of low grade lymphoproliferative malignancies are under investigation.[18]

Interferons in melanoma

Because of their antiproliferative and immunomodulating effects *in vitro*, IFNs have also been used in the treatment of melanoma.[19] Response rates achieved with systemic IFNα, in either high or low dose, in metastatic melanoma were in the range 5–30%, and IFNγ did not appear to be superior.[20,21] Some studies indicate that intralesional injection of IFNα and IFNβ may be effective in cutaneous metastases.[21,22] Recently, encouraging results (30% response) were obtained with a combination of IFNα and DTIC.[21,23,24] Preliminary observations indicate a beneficial effect of IFNα in an adjuvant setting in patients with high risk melanoma.[25] Despite the low efficacy of IFN monotherapy in metastatic disease, several randomized prospective studies are now being performed with IFNs as an adjuvant or in combination with chemotherapy.[23,24]

Interferons in HIV disease

Treatment with IFNα of patients with disseminated AIDS associated Kaposi's sarcoma revealed that high doses resulted in regression in 20–50% of patients.[5,26] However, high dose IFN therapy (up to 4×10^7 U/day) is limited due to the occurrence of severe side-effects, and IFNα in doses less than 2×10^6 u/m² did not prove to be useful.[26] In addition, single cutaneous tumours have been treated successfully with intralesional IFNα.[27]

Interferons in epithelial tumours

Recently, IFNα (1.5×10^6 u three times weekly for 3 weeks) administered intralesionally was introduced for the treatment of actinic keratoses, basal cell carcinoma and squamous cell carcinoma.[28] In most cases the response was evaluated over a 12-week post-treatment period, and in some cases the clearance was confirmed by excisional biopsy specimens. The overall response rate in most trials was 80–100%.[29,30] In contrast, topically applied IFNα was less effective.[31] Similarly, IFNγ proved to be useful in treating basal cell carcinomas.[32] Therefore, in certain subgroups of patients in whom excisions of cancer carries significant functional and surgical risks, intralesional IFN may offer a valuable alternative.

Interferons in atopic dermatitis

Mononuclear cells of patients with atopic dermatitis were found to produce increased levels of interleukin-4 (IL-4), but decreased levels of IFNγ. Moreover, IL-4 levels correlated positively and IFNγ levels negatively with serum IgE levels.[33] In recent studies, subcutaneous injections of IFNγ (50 μg/m² daily for 12 weeks)

resulted in remarkable improvement in skin lesions which was not associated with a decrease in serum IgE levels.[34,35] Although, IFNα treatment inhibited IgE synthesis and improved the cutaneous eruptions in a patient with hyper-IgE syndrome, patients with severe atopic dermatitis do not seem to benefit from IFNα treatment.[5]

Interferons in inflammatory and autoimmune skin diseases

The efficacy of IFNα or IFNγ in psoriasis is controversial. Favourable results have been observed in the treatment of psoriatic arthropathy with IFNγ.[5] In addition, there is clinical evidence that IFN therapy improves the clinical course of certain autoimmune diseases, including rheumatoid arthritis, discoid lupus erythematosus and subacute cutaneous lupus erythematosus.[5,36] Recently, two patients with hepatitis B and concomitant lichen planus were treated with IFNα, which was followed by a total and prolonged disappearance of the lichen planus lesions.[37] However, in three patients, oral lichen planus lesions did not improve on treatment with IFNα ($3–10 \times 10^6$ u three times weekly for 8 weeks) (unpublished observation).

Interferons in disorders of collagen

In vitro, IFNα inhibits collagen and glycosaminoglycan production, normalizes collagenase activity and inhibits fibroblast proliferation.[38] These data suggest that IFNα is a promising candidate for treatment of fibrotic disorders such as keloids or scleroderma. Accordingly, intralesional injections of IFNα (1.5 × 10⁶ U) or IFNγ (50 µg) into progressively enlarging keloids resulted in a significant reduction in their size.[38,39] Treatment of systemic sclerosis with IFNγ resulted in an improvement in the total skin score, whereas dysphagia, Raynaud's phenomenon and cardiac involvement were not affected.[40]

Interferons in other diseases

It has been reported that IFNα blocks the migration of endothelial cells *in vitro* and inhibits angiogenesis in mice.[41] These findings prompted the investigation of the efficacy of subcutaneous injections of IFNα (up to 3 × 10⁶ U/m² per day) for treatment of infants with haemangiomas that failed to respond to corticosteroid treatment. In 18 of the 20 patients the haemangiomas regressed by 50% or more after an average of 7.8 months of treatment.[42] No short-term side-effects have been noticed so far, and the children's growth and development seem to be normal.

A remarkable response to IFNα (5 × 10⁶ U three times weekly) has been observed in one patient with systemic mastocytosis. As is the case with haematological disorders, the time until remission was quite long (2 months).[43] Immunomodulatory agents were used

with moderate success for the treatment of alopecia areata, suggesting a potential therapeutic value of IFNα. However, intralesional IFNα had no significant effect on alopecia areata. Systemic therapy with either IFNα or IFNγ appears to be effective in patients with severe Behçet's disease, as most patients showed rapid clearing of cutaneous and mucosal lesions.[2,5]

Cytokines also play an important role in infectious diseases characterized by granuloma formation, i.e. visceral and cutaneous leishmaniasis and lepromatous leprosy.[44,45] Based on *in vitro* investigations and animal studies, a stimulation of macrophages and an enhancement of the specific T-cell response in experimental leishmaniasis could be demonstrated.[45,46] In a placebo-controlled study, intralesional IFNγ (25 µg four times weekly) injections resulted in complete clearance of four of 13 lesions caused by *Leishmania braziliensis* and nine out of 13 lesions caused by *L. tropica*.[46] In addition, systemic IFNγ (50 µg/m² per day for 4 weeks) proved to be useful in treating cutaneous leishmaniasis.[47] Systemic treatment with IFNγ in combination with pentavalent antimony has been shown to be effective in antimony refractory visceral leishmaniasis as well as in non-pretreated patients.[46]

Side-effects of interferons

Most patients who receive systemic IFN therapy experience flu-like symptoms such as fever, chills, headache, myalgia, and nausea, that respond well to acetaminophen. Haematological changes include leukopenia and thrombocytopenia. Side-effects usually do not exceed World Health Organization grade II and severe changes have been observed only at high doses. Usually the side-effects are rapidly reversible, and no cumulative toxicity has been noted.[5] In some cases, IFN therapy has led to the formation of antinuclear antibodies and to the exacerbation of an underlying autoimmune disease.[48] Another worrying observation during IFN therapy is the development of neutralizing antibodies.[49] This is of importance because the resistance to IFN treatment in hairy cell leukaemia correlates quite well with the development of neutralizing antibodies. However, patients who develop antibodies against recombinant IFNα still respond well to natural IFNα.

Other cytokines

There is only limited experience of the clinical use of other cytokines because many of them were identified quite recently.

Interleukin-2

IL-2 has been shown to be of benefit in the treatment of patients with melanoma, either as monotherapy or in conjunction with adoptive immunotherapy using concurrent transfer of either lymphokine activated killer cells or tumour infiltrating lymphocytes.[50,51] In general, the administration of lymphokine activated killer cells increases the incidence of transient complete remission, but not the overall response.[52] Clinical trials are in progress in which IL-2 is being used in combination with other lymphokines, monoclonal antibodies or chemotherapy.[52] Recent protocols include application of low dose subcutaneous (1.8–18 × 10⁶ U/m² per day) IL-2 and IFNα (3–6 × 10⁶ U/m² three times weekly). Preliminary data indicate that this out-patient regimen can induce objective tumour regressions with low systemic toxicity (World Health Organization grade I and II) in renal cancer and melanoma.[53] There is also recent evidence that IL-2 may be effective in the treatment of haemangioendothelioma. Intralesional administration resulted in disappearance of the tumour, and no recurrence within 1 year was seen.[54] Due to the high doses of IL-2 usually administered, toxicity is severe and mainly related to the vascular leak syndrome.[50,52]

Tumour necrosis factor

Based on its biological activity in animal studies and *in vitro*, tumour necrosis factor α (TNFα) appears to exhibit therapeutic potential.[55] However, TNFα seems to be one of the primary mediators of septic syndrome and shock, and thus its application is limited by severe systemic and local adverse reactions. Upon subcutaneous injection exceeding 150 μg/m² per day, side-effects include severe hypotension, fever, chills, headache, nausea, vomiting, diarrhoea and anorexia.[56] Recently, however, regionally advanced melanoma has been treated with a combination of TNFα (2–4 mg), IFNγ (200 μg) and melphalan (38–120 mg) by isolated limb perfusion. In 23 patients, 21 complete responses and two partial responses were observed.[57] Because of severe toxicity the described regimen is only suitable for local treatment and not for widespread disease.

Promising, but preliminary results have been obtained for the systemic application of TNFα in severe psoriasis. Of five patients treated with TNFα (2–5 × 10⁵ U/m², 3–5 times weekly for 1–3 months) complete clearance of the lesions was observed in three patients and partial clearance in one patient.[58,59]

Colony stimulating factors

Bone marrow toxicity with subsequent susceptibility to infection and haemorrhage is a dose-limiting side-effect of most chemotherapeutic agents. Because of the ability of colony stimulating factors to counteract these complications, many patients undergoing chemotherapy (including those with melanoma) seem to be potential candidates for the application of haematopoietic growth factors. In phase I studies different routes of administration have been used to define the optimum biological dose, the toxicity and the pharmacokinetics of colony stimulating factors. Application of these factors has been demonstrated to result in reduced episodes of infection and in fewer chemotherapy delays.[60-62]

In order to improve the immune function and to overcome chemotherapy related side-effects, colony stimulating factors have been used in HIV-1 infected patients. Granulocyte-macrophage colony stimulating factor (GM-CSF) treatment resulted in a rapid dose-dependent increase in neutrophils and eosinophils as well as in an improvement in neutrophil function.[63,64] Furthermore, in preliminary trials, GM-CSF and granulocyte colony stimulating factor (G-CSF) overcame the myelotoxicity of azidothymidine and ganciclovir therapy.[61,65]

In a recent study GM-CSF was administered subcutaneously to 35 patients with borderline and polar lepromatous forms of leprosy (7.5–45 μg/day for 10 days). There was no evidence of an enhanced cell mediated response to *Mycobacterium lepra* and bacillary numbers remained unchanged. However, enhanced wound healing in 22 of 26 4-mm punch biopsy sites of patients receiving GM-CSF was observed, as compared with the healing time of untreated patients.[66] Recently, it has also been reported that psoriasis in one patient with aplastic anaemia completely cleared after treatment with GM-CSF (3 μg/kg for 3 months).[67]

In contrast to most other biological response modifiers, colony stimulating factors are quite well tolerated. At therapeutic doses the side-effects of GM-CSF include malaise, mild elevation in transaminase levels, bone pain and cutaneous eruptions, all of which are mild to moderate in degree and fully reversible. Recently, the development of a cutaneous maculopapular eruption was reported in patients receiving GM-CSF. G-CSF is well tolerated and, except for bone pain, no significant side-effects have been reported. However, one case of neutrophilic organ infiltration that resembled acute febrile neutrophilic syndrome (Sweet's syndrome) has been described.[5,62,64]

Growth factors

Enhancement of wound healing and reepithelialization is a central problem in the treatment of poorly healing wounds and extensive burn injuries, particularly when autologous donor sites are limited. *In vitro* and *in vivo* studies have demonstrated that keratinocyte derived cytokines and growth factors are involved in pathophysiological mechanisms of wound healing such as local inflammation, reepithelialization and synthesis of matrix proteins.[1]

Recent observations have shown a beneficial effect when either growth factors such as IL-1, epidermal growth factor, transforming growth factor α, fibroblast growth factor, or platelet derived growth factor were applied topically either in ointment or in buffered solution.[5,68] Although these results appear promising, further studies are needed to clarify whether a single growth factor or, more likely, a combination of several mediators will be useful therapeutically in improving wound healing. In addition, transforming growth factor (TGFβ) seems to be essential for hypertrophic scar formation since anti-TGFβ recently has been reported to be effective in controlling scar formation.[69]

Conclusion

The availability of recombinant cytokines in sufficient amounts has allowed the use of these potent regulatory mediators in clinical trials for a variety of diseases. In some instances they already can be regarded as useful therapeutic alternatives. Future prospects include administration of cytokines in combination with standard regimens such as chemotherapy or radiation therapy. Another promising field is cytokine gene therapy. Accordingly, the first clinical trials are being performed using tumour infiltrating lymphocytes transfected with the TNFα gene for treatment of patients with melanoma.[70] Since injection of cytokine secreting tumour cells may generate immunity against unmodified parental tumour cells, clinical trials are being initiated to treat patients having melanoma with their own tumour cells transfected with genes encoding for IL-2 or TNFα.[70] However, much needs to be elucidated with regard to understanding of the complex cytokine interactions in order to obtain a better insight into the role of these mediators in the pathogenesis of disease, and to use them more efficiently in therapy.

References

1   Schwarz T, Luger TA, Pharmacology of cytokines in the skin, In: Muhktar H (ed). *Pharmacology of the skin*. Boca Raton, FL: CRC Press, 1992, pp. 283–314.

2   Stadler R, Mayer da Silva A, Bratzke B et al, Interferons in dermatology, *J Am Acad Dermatol* (1989) 20: 650–6.

3   Levin MJ, Judson FN, Eron L et al, Comparison of intramuscular recombinant alpha interferon (rIFN-2A) with topical acyclovir for the treatment of first-episode herpes genitalis and prevention of recurrences, *Antimicrob Agents Chemother* (1989) 33: 649–52.

4   Duschet P, Schwarz T, Soyer P et al, Treatment of herpes zoster. Recombinant alpha interferon versus acyclovir, *Int J Dermatol* (1988) 27: 193–7.

5   Luger TA, Schwarz T, Therapeutic use of cytokines in dermatology, *J Am Acad Dermatol* (1991) 24: 915–26.

6   Gross G, Ikenberg H, Roussaki A et al, Systemic treatment of condylomata acuminata with recombinant interferon-alpha-2a: low-dose superior to the high-dose regimen, *Chemotherapy* (1986) 32: 537–41.

7   Gross G, Degen W, Hilgarth M et al, Recombinant interferon-gamma in genital warts: results of a multicenter placebo controlled clinical trial, *J Invest Dermatol* (1989) 93: 553.

8   Gross G, Roussaki A, Papendick U, Efficacy of interferons on bowenoid papulosis and other precancerous lesions, *J Invest Dermatol* (1990) 95: 152S–7S.

9   Androphy EJ, Dvoretzky I, Maluish AE et al, Response of warts in epidermo-dysplasia verruciformis to treatment with systemic and intralesional alpha interferon, *J Am Acad Dermatol* (1984) 11: 197–202.

10   Bunn PAJ, Ihde DC, Foon KA, Recombinant interferon alfa-2a, an active agent in advanced cutaneous T-cell lymphomas, *Int J Cancer* (1987) 1 (Suppl.): 9–13.

11   Olsen EA, Rosen ST, Vollmer RT et al, Interferon alfa-2a in the treatment of cutaneous T cell lymphoma, *J Am Acad Dermatol* (1989) 20: 395–407.

12   Vonderheid EC, Thompson R, Smiles KA, Lattanand A, Recombinant interferon alfa-2b in plaque-phase mycosis fungoides. Intralesional and low-dose intramuscular therapy, *Arch Dermatol* (1987) 123: 757–63.

13   Braathen LR, McFadden N, Successful treatment of mycosis fungoides with the combination of etretinate and human recombinant interferon alfa-2a, *J Dermatol Treatment* (1989) 1: 29–32.

14   Thestrup Pedersen K, Hammer R, Kaltoft K et al, Treatment of mycosis fungoides with recombinant interferon-alpha 2a alone and in combination with etretinate, *Br J Dermatol* (1988) 118: 811–18.

15 Knobler R, Trautinger F, Kokoschka EM et al, Possible synergistic effect of interferon alpha-2b and retinoids in the treatment of cutaneous T-cell lymphoma, *J Invest Dermatol* (1989) **93**: 559A.

16 Roenigk HHJ, Kuzel TM, Skoutelis AP et al, Photochemotherapy alone or combined with interferon alpha-2a in the treatment of cutaneous T-cell lymphoma, *J Invest Dermatol* (1990) **95**: 198S–205S.

17 Rook AH, Prystowsky MB, Cassin M et al, Combined therapy for Sezary syndrome with extracorporeal photochemotherapy and low-dose interferon alfa therapy. Clinical, molecular, and immunologic observations, *Arch Dermatol* (1991) **127**: 1535–40.

18 Bunn PAJ, Norris DA, The therapeutic role of interferons and monoclonal antibodies in cutaneous T-cell lymphomas, *J Invest Dermatol* (1990) **95**: 209S–12S.

19 Kirkwood JM, Ernstoff MS, Role of interferons in the therapy of melanoma, *J Invest Dermatol* (1990) **95**: 180S–4S.

20 Landthaler M, Braun Falco O, Adjuvant therapy of high-risk malignant melanoma patients with gamma interferon, *J Am Acad Dermatol* (1989) **20**: 687–8.

21 Stadler R, Garbe C, Interferon therapy in malignant melanoma, *Z Hautkr* (1990) **65**: 504–7.

22 Fierlbeck G, d'Hoedt B, Stroebel W et al, Intraläsionale Therapie von Melanommetastasen mit rekombinanten interferon beta, *Hautarzt* (1992) **43**: 16–21.

23 McLeod GR, Thomson DB, Hersey P, Clinical evaluation of interferons in malignant melanoma, *J Invest Dermatol* (1990) **95**: 185S–7S.

24 Ho VC, Sober AJ, Therapy for cutaneous melanoma: an update, *J Am Acad Dermatol* (1990) **22**: 159–76.

25 Kokoschka EM, Trautinger F, Knobler RM et al, Long-term adjuvant therapy of high-risk malignant melanoma with interferon alpha 2b, *J Invest Dermatol* (1990) **95**: 193S–7S.

26 Real FX, Oettgen HF, Krown SE, Kaposi's sarcoma and the acquired immunodeficiency syndrome: treatment with high and low doses of recombinant leukocyte A interferon, *J Clin Oncol* (1986) **4**: 544–51.

27 Alecu M, Ghyka G, Halalau F et al, Intralesional human leukocyte interferon treatment in the non-AIDS related Kaposi's sarcoma, *Med Int* (1990) **28**: 61–7.

28 Wickramasinghe L, Hindson TC, Wacks H, Treatment of neoplastic skin lesions with intralesional interferon. *J Am Acad Dermatol* (1989) **20**: 71–4.

29 Cornell RC, Greenway HT, Tucker SB et al, Intralesional interferon therapy for basal cell carcinoma, *J Am Acad Dermatol* (1990) **23**: 694–700.

30 Edwards L, Whiting D, Rogers D et al, The effect of an intralesional sustained-released formulation of interferon alpha 2b on basal cell carcinoma, *J Am Acad Dermatol* (1990) **22**: 496–500.

31 Edwards L, Levine N, Smiles KA, The effect of topical interferon alpha 2b on actinic keratoses, *J Dermatol Surg Oncol* (1990) **16**: 446–9.

32 Edwards L, Whiting D, Rogers D et al, The effect of intralesional interferon gamma on basal cell carcinomas, *J Am Acad Dermatol* (1990) **22**: 496–500.

33   Stadler BM, Gauchat JF, Gauchat D et al, Anti-isotype regulation: cytokines and anti-IgE autoantibodies. In: Sorg C (ed). *Cytokines regulating the allergical response*. Basel: Karger, 1989, pp. 37–50.

34   Reinhold U, Wehrmann W, Kukel S, Kreysel HW, Recombinant interferon-gamma in severe atopic dermatitis (letter), *Lancet* (1990) 335: 1282.

35   Hanifin JM, Schneider LC, Leung DYM et al, Recombinant interferon-gamma therapy for atopic dermatitis, *J Invest Dermatol* (1993) 28: 189–97.

36   Lever AM, Brook MG, Yap I, Thomas HC, Treatment of thrombocytopenia with alfa interferon, *Br Med J Clin Res Educ* (1987) 295: 1519–20.

37   Doutre MS, Beylot C, Couzigou P et al, Lichen planus virus C hepatitis: disappearance of the lichen under interferon alpha therapy (letter), *Dermatology* (1992) 184: 229.

38   Granstein RD, Flotte TJ, Amento EP, Interferons and collagen production, *J Invest Dermatol* (1990) 95: 75S–80S.

39   Berman B, Duncan MR, Short-term keloid treatment *in vivo* with human interferon alfa-2b results in a selective and persistent normalization of keloidal fibroblast collagen, glycosaminoglycan, and collagenase production *in vitro*, *J Am Acad Dermatol* (1989) 21: 694–702.

40   Hein R, Behr J, Hündgen M et al, Treatment of systemic sclerosis with gamma-interferon, *Br J Dermatol* (1992) 126: 496–501.

41   Sidky YA, Borden EC, Inhibition of angiogenesis by interferons: effects on tumor- and lymphocyte-induced vascular responses, *Cancer Res* (1987) 47: 5155–61.

42   Ezekowitz RAB, Mulliken JB, Folkman J, Interferon alpha 2a therapy for life-threatening hemangiomas of infancy, *N Engl J Med* (1992) 326: 1456–63.

43   Kluin Nelemans HC, Jansen JH, Breukelman H et al, Response to interferon alfa-2b in a patient with systemic mastocytosis, *N Engl J Med* (1992) 326: 619–23.

44   Nathan CF, Kaplan G, Levis WR et al, Local and systemic effects of intradermal recombinant interferon-gamma in patients with lepromatous leprosy, *N Engl J Med* (1986) 315: 6–15.

45   Badaro R, Falcoff E, Badaro FS et al, Treatment of visceral leishmaniasis with pentavalent antimony and interferon gamma, *N Engl J Med* (1990) 322: 16–21.

46   Harms G, Zwingenberger K, Chehade AK et al, Effects of intradermal gamma-interferon in cutaneous leishmaniasis, *Lancet* (1989) i: 1287–92.

47   Kolde G, Luger TA, Successful treatment of oriental cutaneous leishmaniasis using systemic interferon gamma, *Arch Dermatol Res* (1991) 20: 284A.

48   Conlon KC, Urba WJ, Smith JW et al, Exacerbation of symptoms of autoimmune disease in patients receiving alpha-interferon therapy, *Cancer* (1990) 65: 2237–42.

49   von Wussow P, IFN-treatment of hairy cell leukemia and significance of anti-interferon antibodies, *J Invest Dermatol* (1989) 93: 583A.

50   Lotze MT, Chang AE, Seipp CA et al, High-dose recombinant interleukin 2 in the treatment of patients with disseminated cancer. Responses, treatment-related

morbidity, and histologic findings, *JAMA* (1986) **256**: 3117–24.

51 Rosenberg SA, Packard BS, Aebersold PM et al, Use of tumor-infiltrating lymphocytes and interleukin-2 in the immunotherapy of patients with metastatic melanoma. A preliminary report, *N Engl J Med* (1988) **319**: 1676–80.

52 Lotze MT, Rosenberg SA, The use of lymphokines in therapy. In: Pichler WJ, Stadler BM, Dahinden C (eds). *Progress in allergy and clinical immunology*. Toronto: Hogrefe & Huber, 1989, pp. 529–35.

53 Atzpodien J, Körfer A, Franks CR et al, Home therapy with recombinant interleukin-2 and interferon-α2b in advanced human malignancies, *Lancet* (1990) **335**: 1509–12.

54 Masuzawa M, Asai T, Nishioka K, Nishiyama S, Interleukin-2 therapy for malignant hemangioendothelioma, *J Invest Dermatol* (1989) **93**: 563A.

55 Beutler B, Cerami A, Cachectin (tumor necrosis factor), an endogenous mediator of shock and inflammatory response. In: Oppenheim JJ, Shevach EM (eds). *The role of cells and cytokines in immunity and inflammation*. New York: Oxford University Press, 1990, pp. 226–37.

56 Jakubowski AA, Casper ES, Gabrilove JL et al, Phase I trial of intramuscularly administered tumor necrosis factor in patients with advanced cancer, *J Clin Oncol* (1989) **7**: 298–303.

57 Lienard D, Ewalenko P, Delmotte JJ et al, High-dose recombinant tumor necrosis factor alpha in combination with interferon gamma and melphalan in isolation perfusion of the limbs for melanoma and sarcoma, *J Clin Oncol* (1992) **10**: 52–60.

58 Takematsu H, Ozawa H, Yoshimura T et al, Systemic TNF administration in psoriatic patients: a promising therapeutic modality for severe psoriasis (letter), *Br J Dermatol* (1991) **124**: 209–10.

59 Creaven PJ, Stoll HLJ, Response to tumor necrosis factor in two cases of psoriasis, *J Am Acad Dermatol* (1991) **24**: 735–7.

60 Metcalf D, The colony stimulating factors. Discovery, development, and clinical applications, *Cancer* (1990) **65**: 2185–95.

61 Steward WP, Dunlop DJ, Cassidy J, Dose intensification of chemotherapy in solid tumours with the use of recombinant human granulocyte-macrophage colony stimulating factor, *Behring Inst Mitt* (1991) **90**: 44–9.

62 Lieschke GJ, Burgess AW, Granulocyte colony-stimulating factor and granulocyte-macrophage colony-stimulating factor, *N Engl J Med* (1992) **327**: 99–106.

63 Pluda JM, Yarchoan R, Smith PD et al, Subcutaneous recombinant granulocyte-macrophage colony-stimulating factor used as a single agent and in an alternating regimen with azidothymidine in leukopenic patients with severe human immunodeficiency virus infection, *Blood* (1990) **76**: 463–72.

64 Levine JD, Allan JD, Tessitore JH et al, Recombinant human granulocyte-macrophage colony-stimulating factor ameliorates zidovudine-induced neutropenia in patients with acquired immunodeficiency syndrome (AIDS)/AIDS related complex, *Blood* (1991) **78**: 3148–54.

65 Miles SA, Mitsuyasu RT, Moreno J et al, Combined therapy with recombinant

granulocyte colony-stimulating factor and erythropoietin decreases hematologic toxicity from zidovudine, *Blood* (1991) 77: 2109–17.

66   **Kaplan G, Walsh G, Guido LS et al,** Novel responses of human skin to intradermal recombinant granulocyte/macrophage-colony-stimulating factor: Langerhans cell recruitment, keratinocyte growth, and enhanced wound healing, *J Exp Med* (1992) **175**: 1717–28.

67   **Raychaudhuri SP, Fiore MM,** Clearance of unremitting psoriasis after treatment with granulocyte-macrophage

colony-stimulating factor, *J Am Acad Dermatol* (1992) **27**: 451–2.

68   **Robson MC, Phillips LG, Heggers JP et al,** Clinical studies on growth factors in pressure sores: preliminary report, *Prog Clin Biol Res* (1991) **365**: 95–102.

69   **Shah M, Foreman DM, Ferguson MW,** Control of scarring in adult wounds by neutralising antibody to transforming growth factor beta, *Lancet* (1992) **339**: 213–14.

70   **Miller AD,** Human gene therapy comes of age, *Nature* (1992) **357**: 455–60.

6

New indications for old molecules

Old anti-inflammatory drugs revisited

B. Roger Allen

Introduction

The factors which might stimulate an inflammatory response include physical, chemical, immunological and, of course, infective agents but in many chronic disorders, e.g. rheumatoid disease, psoriasis and atopic dermatitis, the initiating and perpetuating stimuli are unknown.

The classic signs of inflammation—pain, heat, redness and swelling—are characteristically produced by pyogenic infections. Like other normal responses, inflammation is directed towards the restoration of health and is basically a protective and indeed essential response to noxious stimuli; it confines and repairs injury. If the stimulus is transient and localized, for example from a burn, there is steady progress from the acute to the resolving phase with the operation of normal negative feedback mechanisms, most of which are only inadequately understood, and the inflammation resolves. Sometimes the response is too severe, too prolonged or inappropriately stimulated; under which circumstances tissue damage may result in morbidity and loss of function. It is the body's own defences which cause the symptoms of inflammation and it is the inflammatory response which eventually causes damage.

At the pathophysiological level, inflammation results in small vessel dilatation with increased blood flow, extravasation of fluid into the tissues and leukocyte margination and migration through the postcapillary venule.

What is clearly apparent is that the clinical and histological manifestations of the dermatoses labelled 'inflammatory' vary considerably. The pain of a pyogenic folliculitis, the intense irritation of dermatitis and the erythema and scaling of active psoriasis are obviously features of differing processes. This has resulted in a broadening of our concept of what constitutes inflammation and much research over the past 50 years or more has been directed towards determining the nature and properties of individual inflammatory components.

Broadly the inflammatory response is seen to consist of two components, cellular and soluble (Table 6.1), although the two are interactive and inextricably linked with, for example, migratory cells both reacting to and producing soluble mediators, such as cytokines, and eicosanoids. The release of mediators is sequential, as is the nature of the cellular infiltrate. In the earliest stages after injury histamine

Table 6.1 Components of inflammatory responses in the skin

Cellular

CIRCULATING CELLS	TISSUE CELLS
Phagocytic	Endothelial cells
Neutrophils	Fibroblasts
Eosinophils	Mast cells
Monocytes	Keratinocytes
Lymphocytes	
Platelets	

Soluble

LIPID DERIVED	AMINO ACID DERIVED
Eicosanoids	Histamine
Prostaglandins	Serotonin
Leukotrienes	Immunoglobulins
Thromboxanes	Complement
Platelet Activating	Contact
Factors	activation system
	Cytokines
	Adhesion
	molecules

MISCELLANEOUS
Calcium ions
Free radicals

and 5-hydroxytryptamine predominate and there is vasodilatation and increased vascular permeability. The interaction between the endothelial cells and circulating polymorphonuclear leucocytes at this stage has been clearly shown by the work of Wedmore and Williams[1] who demonstrated that, in the absence of circulating polymorphonuclear leucocytes, vasodilatation was not accompanied by plasma leakage. This is supported at the clinical level by the symptoms displayed in patients with defects in different components of the inflammatory response. Patients with leukocyte adhesion deficiency[2] who lack the necessary intercellular adhesion molecules which allow circulating leukocytes to marginate and migrate through the postcapillary venule wall have a defective inflammatory response, despite high numbers of circulating leukocytes, as do those with the Chediak–Higashi and Job syndromes where the response of leukocytes to chemotactic stimuli is defective. Conversely, patients with chronic granulomatous disease, where excessive numbers of leukocytes migrate but are defective in oxygen dependent killing mechanisms, produce inflammatory responses which are severe and prolonged.

Anti-inflammatory therapy is aimed at breaking the chain of events in an unwanted inflammatory response at a strategic point by competitive inhibition of a mediator or inhibition of an enzyme vital to its formation, or the destruction of cells by cytotoxic activity, or altering their mobility by impairing or enhancing their ability to respond to chemokinetic or chemotactic stimuli. It is important that any effect achieved is only temporary or partial and that it is controlled and reversible or normal inflammatory responses to injury may be impaired with damaging consequences. It is a sobering thought that almost all the therapeutic advances in the treatment of inflammatory skin disease have been made by serendipity associated with careful clinical observation, rather than by directed research.

The individual components of the inflammatory chain, as outlined in Table 6.1, are all potentially open to drug manipulation, but it would probably be a mistake, from the therapeutic point of view, to concentrate on targeting individual mediators in isolation: the ultimate test of an anti-inflammatory drug is not whether it is a potent inhibitor of one particular enzyme but whether it improves a clinical condition.

Drugs affecting lipid mediators of inflammation

Until the description of a lipid soluble factor in human seminal fluid which caused profound hypotension in rabbits,[3] most inflammatory mediators were believed to be related to water soluble amino acids. The first prostaglandins were isolated in 1957,[4] thromboxane was isolated in 1975[5] and slow reacting substances of anaphylaxis (SRS-A) were identified as lipid mediators in 1978.[6] In 1979, Borgeat and Samuelsson[7,8] described the generation of several dihydroxy derivatives of arachidonic acid following incubation with isolated rabbit polymorphonuclear leucocytes. With the demonstration by Vane[9] that non-steroidal anti-inflammatory drugs (NSAIDs) act through their ability to block prostaglandin synthetase (cyclo-oxygenase), an *in vitro* model with predictive value for assessing anti-inflammatory activity became available. As a result, a considerable number of NSAIDs have been developed which vary little in their therapeutic effects. That these compounds do indeed exert their effect through inhibition of prostaglandin formation is supported by the fact that cyclo-oxygenase is inhibited by concentrations (0.1–10 µg) which are comparable to achievable therapeutic levels and by the good correlation between cyclo-oxygenase inhibition and anti-inflammatory activity. There are anomalies, and the ill-fated drug benoxaprofen, for example, had an anti-inflammatory effect which was disproportionately greater than its ability to inhibit prostaglandin synthesis would have predicted.[10] The classical anti-inflammatory drugs vary considerably in their chemical structure, although most are weak organic acids. The major groups and some examples are shown in Table 6.2.

Salicylates

Salicylate-containing plant extracts have been used in Western medicine since before the time of Hippocrates[11] and acetylsalicylic acid (Aspirin) was one of the first drugs to be synthesized.

Table 6.2   Chemical groups of non-steroidal anti-inflammatory drugs

Salicylates	Aspirin
	Diflunisal
	Sodium salicylate
Indoleacetic acids	Indomethacin
Sulindac	
Pyrazoles	Phenylbutazone
	Oxyphenbutazone
Propionic acids	Benoxaprofen
	Ibuprofen
	Ketoprofen
Fenamates	Meclofenamate
	Mefenamic acid
Oxicams	Piroxicam
Naphthaleneacetic acids	Naproxen

In the biphasic inflammatory response seen in the rat paw as a result of injections of carrageenan (sulphurated polysaccharides extracted from the Irish moss *Chondrus crispus*) initial swelling is accompanied by the release of histamine and serotonin. After 3 h a second phase of more prolonged swelling develops and this is accompanied by the release of eicosanoids and a marked polymorphonuclear leukocyte and platelet infiltrate. It is this second phase which is inhibited by aspirin and other NSAIDs. Aspirin inhibits prostaglandin synthesis by the irreversible acetylation of the cyclo-oxygenase enzyme.[12] It is thus different in its mode of action from other cyclo-oxygenase inhibitors which inhibit the enzyme in a rapidly reversible manner.

Salicylic acid has been widely used in dermatological preparations in concentrations of 0.5–50% as a keratolytic and also to enhance the efficacy of topical steroids.[13] Salicylism through percutaneous absorption is a risk where salicylic acid is applied to large areas of the body surface, but any local anti-inflammatory effect is slight. However pretreatment with oral aspirin can greatly reduce the inflammation and prostaglandin formation induced by topical application to the skin of tetrahydrofurfuryl nicotinate.[14] Methylsalicylate, widely used as a local counter-irritant, has no anti-inflammatory properties. It behaves as a prodrug and after absorption is rapidly hydrolysed to salicylic acid.

Indomethacin and cyclo-oxygenase inhibitors

Indomethacin was introduced as an alternative to salicylates and the unacceptably toxic drug phenylbuta-zone in 1963. Vane[9] showed that it reduced prostaglandin formation by virtue of its cyclo-oxygenase inhibiting property and it became the standard by which other NSAIDs were assessed.

Prostaglandins, particularly prosta-glandin E_2 (PGE$_2$), have been impli-cated in the erythema of allergic contact dermatitis,[15] ultraviolet erythema[16,17] and possibly psoriasis. Indomethacin applied topically will suppress the formation of PGE$_2$ in ultraviolet irradiated skin, although the inhibition of erythema is less than complete.[18] However, despite the fact that indomethacin has been available for a quarter of a century, it has not earned a regular place in the therapy of skin disease. Although increased levels of PGE$_2$ have been detected in psori-atic lesional skin,[19] there is no evidence that indomethacin has a beneficial effect on psoriasis,[20] and indeed there are reports that it can worsen the condition when administered either systemically or topically.[21,22] It is not clear whether the adverse effect of indomethacin is due to inhibition of PGE$_2$ formation, with resulting loss of a normal negative feedback mecha-nism, for example, on interleukin-1 production, or to diversion of liberated arachidonic acid down an alternative lipoxygenase pathway with an increased production of lipoxygenase products. Certainly the level of 12-lipoxygenase products generated *in vitro* by isolated peripheral leukocytes rises with indomethacin treatment, but this by itself is unlikely to be the cause of the deterioration since benoxapro-fen, which improves psoriasis, has the same effect.[23]

Dual inhibitors

Following the discovery of the lipoxy-genase pathways of arachidonic acid metabolism came the suggestion that inhibition of lipoxygenases, in addition to cyclo-oxygenase, could be of additional benefit in the treatment of inflammatory diseases,[24] and so-called 'dual inhibitors' have been sought. Up to the present time no systemically administered drug has been licensed for use in humans, due either to toxicity, poor absorption or too rapid metabolism.

The compound which has been most studied *in vitro* and in animals is the aminopyrazaline BW 755C (3-amino-1-(*m*-(trifluromethyl)phenyl)pyrazoline). This phenidone derivative produces a dose-dependent reduction in carrageenin-induced oedema but, unlike indomethacin, it reduces the total number of leukocytes in the inflammatory infiltrate as well.[25] Although the drug has not been used in humans, a similar reduction in the cellular infiltrate was found using the non-steroidal drug benoxaprofen,[26] which in clinical use proved to have a different spectrum of activity from other NSAIDs with, for example, a striking effect on the lesions of psoriasis.[27] Benoxaprofen inhibited the production of 5-lipoxygenase products from rabbit peritoneal cells stimulated with calcium ionophore A23187[28] and also of leukotrienes released by anaphylactic reactions from guinea-pig lungs.[29] However, doubt has been cast on whether inhibition of 5-lipoxygenase accounts for the differences between benoxaprofen and other NSAIDs[30] and studies on the purified 5-lipoxygenase enzyme have failed to demonstrate an effect.[31] Nevertheless, a reduction in the cellular content of inflammatory infiltrates, however achieved, may be a valuable measure of an anti-inflammatory drug with additional properties, whether or not it is acting as a 'dual inhibitor' at the enzymatic level. Other suggested mechanisms to explain the unique effects of benoxaprofen include a pro-oxidant effect,[32,33] the stimulation of interleukin-1 production,[34] a property it may share with retinoids, which again may be through a pro-oxidant effect, and the inhibition of the adhesion of monocytes to endothelial cells.[35] We have been unable to confirm this latter effect,[36] but have noted an effect on 12,20-di-hydroxyeicosatetraenoic (HETE) acid production in mixed peripheral leukocytes treated with benoxaprofen.[23] This dihydroxy derivative of arachidonic acid is believed to be formed by the action of polymorphonuclear leukocyte Ω-hydroxylase on platelet produced 12-HETE. Levels are increased in cells from psoriatics and the levels are reduced by benoxaprofen, despite a rise in 12-HETE.

The significance of these observations has yet to be elucidated. Of great importance in considering the action of such drugs is the fact that many of the components of the inflammatory chain (Table 6.1) were not discovered at the time that the basic research on them was being carried out. A fresh assessment may be necessary in order to clarify their action.

The enzyme 5-lipoxygenase catalyses the first two steps in the conversion of arachidonic acid to the biologically active leukotrienes.[37] It is therefore pivotal in the formation of both SRS-A activity resulting from sulphidopeptide leukotriene (LTC_4, LTD_4, LTE_4) formation and of chemotactic LTB_4. Current interest in the enzyme as a target both for research, to help our understanding of the natural control mechanisms of eicosanoid metabolism, and for the development of inhibitors which might be useful therapeutically, is understandable and logical. Progress in both areas has been hampered by the lack of an adequate inflammatory model in which 5-lipoxygenase products can be proved to be essential. Arachidonic acid or calcium ionophore A23187 induced inflammation of the mouse ear is a widely used bioassay system, although many test substances which have 5-lipoxygenase inhibitory properties *in vitro* fail to influence the inflammation *in vivo*, whereas drugs with a wide variety of different pharmacological actions will cause suppression.[38]

Antagonists of the sulphidopeptide leukotrienes

The sulphidopeptide leukotrienes may be of importance in inflammatory skin disease. Experimentally, in human skin, the local injection of LTC_4 and LTD_4 produces a weal and persistent flare[39] and an increase in microvascular blood flow.[40] Increased levels of LTC_4 have been detected in involved psoriatic skin[41] and LTC_4 and LTD_4 have been shown to be capable of causing epidermal cell proliferation.[42] Receptor antagonists might therefore prove valuable in the treatment of inflammatory skin disease. Studies using specific antagonists which are currently undergoing assessment in other conditions are awaited with interest.[43]

Conclusions

Our understanding of the inflammatory process is steadily increasing and it is easy to overlook the fact that many older drugs were intensively studied and developed at a time when many of the mediators of which we are now aware had not been described. Studies on the effects such drugs have on these mediators are consequently lacking. Benoxaprofen has been discussed above, but other drugs are known to have had some unusual effects. Levamisole was extremely fashionable a few years ago as a stimulant of the immune response[44] and, whilst it is known to be a stimulant of chemokinesis,[45] it may have other properties. Recently, it has been shown to have steroid sparing properties in children with glomerulonephritis[46] and the same might apply to skin disease. Thalidomide[47] and dapsone might also justify further studies in the light of our current understanding of the inflammatory response, as may heparin which has for many years been known to benefit dermatitis herpetiformis.[48]

References

1   Wedmore CV, Williams TJ, Control of vascular permeability by polymorphonuclear leukocytes in inflammation, *Nature* (1981) **289**: 646.

2   Crowley CA, Curnette JT, Rosin RE et al, An inherited abnormality of neutrophil adhesion: its genetic transmission and association with a missing protein, *N Eng J Med* (1980) **302**: 1163–8.

3   von Euler US, *Arch Exp Pathol Pharmakol* (1934) **17**: 578–84.

4   Bergstrom S, Sjovali J, *Acta Chem Scand* (1957) **11**: 1086.

5   Hamberg M, Svensson J, Samuelsson B, Thromboxanes: a new group of biologically active compounds derived from prostaglandin endoperoxides, *Proc Natl Acad Sci USA* (1975) **72**: 2994–8.

6   Morris HR, Taylor GW, Piper PJ et al, Slow-reacting substance of anaphylaxis: purification and characterisation, *FEBS Lett* (1978) **87**: 203–6.

7   Borgeat P, Samuelsson B, Transformation of arachidonic acid by rabbit polymorphonuclear leukocytes, *J Biol Chem* (1979) **254**: 2643–6.

8   Borgeat P, Samuelsson B, Metabolism of arachidonic acid in polymorphonuclear leukocytes, *J Biol Chem* (1979) **254**: 7865–9.

9   Vane JR, Inhibition of prostaglandin synthesis as a mechanism of action for aspirin like drugs, *Nature (New Biol)* (1971) **231**: 232.

10   Cashin CH, Dawson W, Kitchen EA, The pharmacology of benoxaprofen, *J Pharm Pharmacol* (1977) **29**: 330.

11   Rainsford KD, *Aspirin and the salicylates*. London: Butterworths, 1984.

12   Roth GJ, Stanford N, Majerus PW, Acetylation of prostaglandin synthetase by aspirin, *Proc Natl Acad Sci USA* (1975) **72**: 3073.

13   Elie R, Durocher L-P, Kavalec EC, Effect of salicylic acid on the activity of betamethasone-17,21-dipropionate in the treatment of erythematous squamous dermatoses, *J Int Med Res* (1983) **11**: 108–12.

14   Plummer NA, Hensby CN, Kobza Black A, Greaves MW, Prostaglandin activity in sustained inflammation of human skin before and after aspirin, *Clin Sci Mol Med* (1977) **52**: 615–20.

15   Barr RM, Brain S, Camp RDR et al, Human allergic and irritant contact dermatitis; levels of arachidonic acid and its metabolites in involved skin, *Br J Dermatol* (1984) **111**: 23–8.

16   Kobza Black A, Fincham N, Greaves MW, Hensby CN, Time course changes in levels of arachidonic acid and prostaglandins D2 E2 and F2 in human skin following ultraviolet B irradiation, *Br J Pharmacol* (1980) **10**: 453–7.

17   Snyder DS, Eaglstein WH, Topical indomethacin and sunburn, *Br J Dermatol* (1974) **90**: 91–3.

18   Kobza Black A, Greaves MW, Hensby CN et al, Effects of indomethacin on prostaglandins E_2 F_{2a} and arachidonic acid in human skin 24 h after UVB and UVC irradiation, *Br J Pharmacol* (1978) **6**: 261–6.

19   Hammarstrom S, Hamberg M, Samuelsson B et al, Increased concentrations of non-esterified arachidonic acid, 12-L-hydroxy-5,8,12,14-eicosatetraenoic acid,

prostaglandin E_2 and prostaglandin F_2 in epidermis of psoriasis, *Proc Natl Acad Sci USA* (1975) 72: 5130–5.

20 Kern AB, Indomethacin for psoriasis, *Arch Dermatol* (1966) 93: 239–40.

21 Katamaya H, Kawada A, Exacerbation of psoriasis induced by indomethacin, *J Dermatol* (1981) 8: 323–7.

22 Ellis CN, Fallon JD, Heezen JL, Voorhees JJ, Topical indomethacin exacerbates the lesions of psoriasis, *Clin Res* (1983) 31 (2): 564A.

23 Maurice PDL, Allen BR, Heptinstall S, Bather PC, Arachidonic acid metabolism by peripheral blood cells in psoriasis, *Br J Dermatol* (1986) 114: 553–66.

24 Higgs GA, Flower RJ, Anti-inflammatory drugs and the inhibition of arachidonate lipoxygenase. In: Piper PJ (ed). *SRS-A and leukotrienes.* New York: Wiley, 1981.

25 Higgs GA, Eakins KE, Mugridge KG et al, The effects of non-steroidal anti-inflammatory drugs on leukocyte migration in carrageenin induced inflammation, *Eur J Pharmacol* (1980) 66: 81–6.

26 Meacock SCR, Kitchen EA, Effects of the non-steroidal anti inflammatory drug benoxaprofen on leukocyte migration, *J Pharm Pharmacol* (1979) 31: 366–70.

27 Allen BR, Littlewood SM, Benoxaprofen: effect on cutaneous lesions in psoriasis, *Br Med J* (1982) 285: 1241.

28 Walker JR, Dawson W, Inhibition of rabbit polymorphonuclear lipoxygenase activity by benoxaprofen, *J Pharm Pharmacol* (1979) 31: 778–80.

29 Boot JR, Sweatman WJF, Cox BA et al, The anti-allergic effects of benoxaprofen, a lipoxygenase inhibitor, *Int Arch Allergy Appl Immunol* (1982) 67: 340–3.

30 Salmon JA, Tilling LC, Moncada S, Evaluation of inhibitors of eicosanoid synthesis in leukocytes: possible pitfalls of using the calcium ionophore A23187 to stimulate 5-lipoxygenase, *Prostaglandins* (1985) 29: 377–85.

31 Salmon JA, Higgs GA, Tilling L et al, Mode of action of benoxaprofen, *Lancet* (1984) i: 848.

32 Anderson R, Lukey PT, Naude SPE, Joone G, Benoxaprofen: a pro-oxidant anti-inflammatory drug, *Agents Actions* (1984) 14: 238.

33 Anderson R, Eftychis HA, Potentiation of the generation of reactive oxidants by human phagocytes during exposure to benoxaprofen and ultraviolet radiation *in vitro, Br J Dermatol* (1986) 115: 285–95.

34 Rainsford KD, *Int J Tissue Reactions* (1985) VII: 123.

35 Brown KA, Ferrie J, Wilbourn B, Dumonde DC, Benoxaprofen, a potent inhibitor of monocyte/endothelial cell interaction, *Lancet* (1984) ii: 643.

36 Barkley ASJ, Bather PC, Allen BR, Retinoids enhance monocyte/endothelial cell interaction, *J Invest Dermatol* (1987) 89: 320.

37 Taylor GW, Morris HR, Lipoxygenase pathways, *Br Med Bull* (1983) 39: 219–22.

38 Chang J, Doherty MS, Models of inflammatory disease and eicosanoid activities. In: Lewis A, Ackerman N, Otterness I (eds). *Advances in inflammation research. Vol. 12: New perspectives in*

anti-inflammatory therapies. New York: Raven Press, 1988.

39   Soter NA, Lewis RA, Corey EJ, Austen KF, Local effects of synthetic leukotrienes (LTC$_4$, LTD$_4$, LTE$_4$, and LTB$_4$) in human skin, *J Invest Dermatol* (1983) **80**: 115–19.

40   Bisgaard H, Kristensen J, Sondergaard J, The effect of leukotriene C$_4$ and D$_4$ on cutaneous blood flow in humans, *Prostaglandins* (1982) **23**: 797–801.

41   Brain SD, Camp RD, Charleson S et al, The release of LTC$_4$-like material from the involved lesional skin in psoriasis, *Br J Pharmacol* (1983) **17**: 6501.

42   Kragballe K, Voorhees JJ, Modulation of epidermal cell division and growth by oxygenation products of arachidonic acid, *J Allergy Clin Immunol* (1984) **74**: 426–9.

43   Taylor IK, O'Shaugnessy KM, Fuller RW, Dollery CT, Effect of cysteinyl-leukotriene receptor antagonist ICI 204.219 on allergen-induced bronchoconstriction and airway hyperactivity in atopic subjects, *Lancet* (1991) **337**: 690–4.

44   Gilman AG, Goodman LS, Rall TW, Murad F (eds), *Goodman and Gilman's pharmacological basis of therapeutics,* New York: MacMillan, 1985, 7th edn, p. 1012.

45   Wright DG, Kirkpatrick CH, Gallin JI, Effects of levamisole on normal and abnormal leukocyte locomotion, *J Clin Invest* (1977) **59**: 941–50.

46   British Association for Paediatric Nephrology, Levamisole for corticosteroid-dependent nephrotic syndrome in childhood, *Lancet* (1991) **337**: 1555–7.

47   Koch HP, Thalidomide and cogeners as anti-inflammatory agents. In: Ellis GP, West GB (eds). *Progress in Medicinal Chemistry 22,* Amsterdam, Elsevier, 1985.

48   Alexander JO'D, *Dermatitis herpetiformis,* London: W.B. Saunders, 1975.

7

Traditional Chinese medicine for atopic eczema

John Harper

History and philosophy of traditional Chinese medicine

Traditional Chinese medicine (TCM) is based on a philosophy which has evolved over a period of thousands of years. Basic to this philosophy is the concept of harmony with Nature, with the main organs of the body and with mental and physical conditions. Each of the five major organs (heart, lungs, liver, spleen and kidneys) are linked with elements (fire, metal, wood, earth and water), cosmic phases (e.g. summer and spring), tastes, colours and climates (hot, dry, windy, damp and cold).

TCM dates back to the 5th century B.C. and one of the more famous medical works *Nei Jing* (The Yellow Emperor's Internal Classic) was compiled some three centuries B.C.

From these early times, hundreds of prescriptions were available and many of them used plant materials.

In TCM, eczema is associated with the lungs and also with the heart, blood and stomach. It is believed that weeping eczema is caused by 'damp heat' and results in discharge, hotness and itching. Dry eczema is attributed to 'heat in the blood', whereas skin eruptions are said to be caused by 'wind'. Eczema caused by wind may be treated by herbs such as *Paeonia*, *Rehmannia*, *Schizonepeta* and *Ledebouriella*.

Chinese prescriptions contain more than a single herb and each prescription is designed for an individual patient. In each prescription there is a chief herb or 'emperor' and other herbs which are considered in rank order as 'chief minister', 'ministers', 'senior officers' and 'junior officers'.

Clinical studies

It is difficult for Western doctors to understand this approach to treatment, but the therapeutic effectiveness of this type of treatment was brought to my attention by a Chinese practitioner in London, Dr Ding-Hui Luo, who had been successfully treating a large number of children with individual formulations of a 'tea' prepared from selected herbs. The response to treatment was undoubtedly impressive, with a noticeable improvement in the skin condition and a reduction of pruritus, often within the first week, in children in whom conventional 'Western' treatments had failed. This observation prompted our original publication in the *Lancet* in 1990.[1]

In collaboration with Prof. J.D. Phillipson at The School of Pharmacy, University of London, and Dr S.J. Corne at Stiefel Laboratories, International Division, Wooburn Green, UK, we set out to investigate scientifically these plant materials. Dr Luo provided me with details of her prescriptions and we chose to look at the plants most commonly used by her in the treatment of eczema.

Our early attempts to identify one or more active agents within the TCM eczema treatment were guided by anti-inflammatory tests in mice. Based on this work we embarked on a series of clinical pilot studies. First we used a standardized mixture of four plants: *Radix ledebouriellae*, *Radix rehmannia*, *Radix paeoniae rubra* and *Radix glycyrrhizae*. Eight patients participated (aged 2–12 years). Treatment was assessed over a 3-week period. Six patients completed the study. All six improved, especially as far as loss of sleep and itch was concerned. Next, three more plants, *Rhizoma smilacis glabrae*, *Cortex dictamni radicis* and *Fructus tribuli*, were added to the mixture in an attempt to produce an enhanced clinical effect. The same protocol was applied. In all six patients who participated there was a significant improvement in the skin condition as well as in loss of sleep and itch.

By this stage other research workers had established an interest in this field. A placebo-controlled double-blind trial of a specific formulation of plant materials in prepared 'tea bags' (Formula PSE 101, Phytopharm, Brough, UK) was undertaken in children with severe, widespread eczema.[2] The plant materials used were: *Ledebouriella seseloides*, *Potentilla chinensis*, *Akebia clematidis*, *Rehmannia glutinosa*, *Paeonia lactiflora*, *Lophatherum gracile*, *Dictamnus dasycarpus*, *Tribulus terrestris*, *Glycyrrhiza uralensis* and *Schizonepeta tenuifolia*. The placebo was a mixture of inert plant materials of similar appearance, taste and smell, but with no known benefit in atopic eczema. The study in 47 children showed a significant beneficial response for the active treatment compared with placebo in children with severe widespread non-exudative atopic eczema. A similar study in adults using the same 'tea bags' also showed a significant beneficial response.[3]

As an extension to this work, a standardized dried extract of the same herbs (Formula PSE 201, Phytopharm, Brough, UK) demonstrated a beneficial effect in 21 patients who completed an open pilot study of 2 months treatment (H Goodyear and JI Harper, personal communication).

The major difficulty with all these treatments has to date been their unpleasant taste, and this aspect has now been addressed with the development of a new palatable preparation. A placebo-controlled double-blind multi-centre study of this product is planned.

Pharmacology and toxicology

This combination of plant materials contains a veritable pot-pourri of chemicals, including alkaloids, chromones, coumarins, flavenoids, glycosides, iridoids, monoterpenes, saponins, steroids, tannins, triterpenoids and volatile oils. Such compounds are known as secondary compounds and are the expression of the major biosynthetic pathways in plants being derived via acetate and shikimate pathways. Some of these compounds may have direct pharmacological actions at specific sites or may act as immunomodulating agents.

Our early attempts to identify a single active herb within the TCM eczema treatment were guided by anti-inflammatory tests in mice. It was shown that some of the plant materials possess anti-inflammatory activity, as assessed by abdominal constriction tests in mice, and that some have a sedative effect. Transferring this information into clinical treatment showed that the dramatic effects against eczema were due to the 10 herbs in combination and that this effect could not be reproduced clinically by a lesser number of herbs chosen on the basis of pharmacological tests in mice.

Until more is known about the chemical nature and actions of these compounds, there must remain an awareness for possible long-term toxicity. There have been reports of hepatotoxicity associated with Chinese herbal remedies.[4-6] Careful clinical monitoring is therefore essential.

Summary

Perhaps we should not be too surprised that TCM utilizes a mixture of plant materials in order to treat eczema, when we compare 'Western' treatments which include emollients, topical steroids, antibiotics and antihistamines. We have been impressed by the therapeutic benefit in children with severe atopic eczema; for specific types or patterns of eczema the TCM preparation would appear to be clinically superior to 'Western' treatment in selected patients. It is our hope that new and better standardized treatments for atopic eczema will be developed from these plant materials.

References

1 Harper JI, Yang S-L, Evans FJ, Phillipson JD, Chinese herbs for eczema, *Lancet* (1990) **335**: 795.

2 Sheehan MP, Atherton DJ, A controlled trial of traditional Chinese medicinal plants in widespread non-exudative atopic eczema, *Br J Dermatol* (1992) **126**: 179–84.

3 Sheehan MP, Rustin MHA, Atherton DJ et al, Efficacy of traditional Chinese herbal therapy in adult atopic dermatitis, *Lancet* (1992) **340**: 13–17.

4 Davies EG, Pollock I, Steel HM, Chinese herbs for eczema, *Lancet* (1990) **336**: 177.

5 **Graham-Brown R,** Toxicity of Chinese herbal remedies, *Lancet* (1992) **340:** 673.

6 **Mostefa-Kara N, Pauwels A, Pinus E et al,** Fatal hepatitis after herbal tea, *Lancet* (1992) **340:** 674.

8

Anti-parasitic agents

D. Anthony Burns

Head louse infection

For several years two insecticides, malathion and carbaryl, have provided the mainstay of treatment for head louse infection in the UK. The former was introduced in 1971, and largely replaced the use of γ-benzene hexachloride (lindane). At the time when malathion was introduced, there was evidence of resistance of head lice to lindane. A decade later, carbaryl became available for clinical use. Subsequently, it became the policy in most health districts to alternate the use of these two insecticides every 3 years, in order to reduce the possibility of the emergence of lice resistant to malathion and carbaryl. Both insecticides are very effective pediculicides, rapidly killing adult lice, and they also have good ovicidal activity (60–80%). Malathion is adsorbed on keratin, and the residual insecticidal activity which results is said to confer protection against reinfection for 6 weeks. Carbaryl, however, does not have any residual activity. It is recommended that these insecticides should be used twice, with the two treatments separated by an interval of 7–10 days. They have proved extremely useful in head louse control for several years.

More recently, the synthetic pyrethroids, a new group of insecticides with potent pediculicidal activity, have been introduced for the treatment of head lice.

Synthetic pyrethroids

Synthetic pyrethroids were developed from pyrethrins, naturally occurring insecticides derived from plants of the genus *Chrysanthemum*. Pediculicides containing natural pyrethrins and the synergist piperonyl butoxide have been used since 1950. Natural pyrethrins are unstable in heat and sunlight, but the synthetic pyrethroids are thermostable and photostable, whilst retaining high insecticidal activity, and having low mammalian toxicity. They are rapidly biodegraded. In these times of greater awareness of environmental issues, the synthetic pyrethroids are approaching the ideal of a 'green' insecticide. The first light-stable synthetic pyrethroid to be developed was permethrin.

In 1986, Taplin and his colleagues reported the results of a trial in which a 1% permethrin creme rinse ('Nix') was used to treat head lice. The study was carried out in the Republic of Panama. Fourteen days after a single treatment with the permethrin product, 97% of those treated were free of lice. Subsequent studies have confirmed the pediculicidal efficacy of permethrin.

It was not until relatively recently that this permethrin creme rinse product became available in the UK, under the trade name 'Lyclear Creme Rinse'. The hair is first washed with an ordinary proprietary shampoo; the creme rinse is then applied for 10 min in sufficient quantity to saturate the hair and scalp, and subsequently removed by rinsing with water. A residue of permethrin remains on the hair, and confers a protective effect against reinfection for several weeks.

Phenothrin is another synthetic pyrethroid which has recently been introduced for the treatment of head lice, and is available in shampoo and lotion formulations — 'Full Marks' shampoo, and 'Full Marks' lotion. The shampoo preparation has been temporarily withdrawn because of eye irritancy.

Although the synthetic pyrethroids are excellent pediculicides, they are not completely ovicidal. It is preferable, therefore, to repeat treatment after an interval of 7–10 days.

Head louse repellent

Head louse infection is a common problem, and it is not unusual for children to suffer repeated reinfection if they are in an environment where they are in contact with a large number of affected individuals. Anxious parents will sometimes resort to repeated 'prophylactic' use of insecticides, a misuse which should be discouraged. In these circumstances a louse repellent is preferable, and such a preparation has recently become available. 'Rappell' is a head louse repellent the active component of which is piperonal, a plant-derived compound which is already widely used as a food flavouring agent and fragrance. In studies at the Medical Entomology Centre at the University of Cambridge, it was discovered that lice, in contrast with their human hosts, did not appear to find piperonal in the least appetizing. When exposed to piperonal on filter-paper discs lice were very positive in their movement away from this agent. The reason for this repellent effect is not known.

'Rappell' is marketed in a pump spray, and has quite a pleasant aroma. Used once daily on the hair, it is said to be an effective louse repellent.

Clothing louse infection

In developed countries clothing louse infection is usually only encountered in tramps and down-and-outs, whose clothing is rarely removed or cleaned. High temperature laundering of clothing, tumble-drying, and dry-cleaning will kill lice and eggs. However, in many parts of the world where there is widespread poverty, clothing louse infection is common, and presents a significant health hazard in view of the ability of these parasites to transmit typhus and louse-borne relapsing fever. In these circumstances louse control involves the use of dusting powders on the clothing. In the 1940s, DDT was employed for this purpose, but this was superceded by γ-benzene hexachloride (lindane) following the emergence of DDT-resistant lice. Subsequent reports of resistance to lindane led to the development and use of malathion powder, and more recently permethrin powder has been employed for clothing louse control.

Crab louse infection

Crab louse infection is a common problem among sexually active young adults. Preparations containing lindane or malathion are the mainstay of treatment for crab louse infection in the UK, but synergized pyrethrins and pyrethroids are also effective against these lice. However, as the ovicidal activity of these insecticides is not complete, they should all be used on two occasions, separated by an interval of 7–10 days. The majority of practitioners in the UK treat patients with Quellada lotion (lindane) or Derbac-M liquid (malathion). These are both water-based preparations, and their use is preferable to preparations with an alcohol base, which are irritant to the scrotum.

The crab louse will colonize the scalp margins, eyelashes, beard, axillary hair, pubic hair, and hairs on the trunk and limbs. Hence, all these areas should be treated to ensure complete eradication of the infection.

Eyelash infection

Petrolatum and physostigmine eye ointment have been popular remedies for crab lice on the eyelashes, but both require several applications over a number of days if they are to eradicate the infection. It is preferable to employ a water-based insecticide such as Quellada lotion or Derbac-M liquid. This can be smeared on the eyelids and lashes, and two applications separated by an interval of 7–10 days are usually effective. Alcohol-based preparations should not be used as they are irritant to the eyes.

Scabies

There have been many remedies for scabies in the past. Sulphur preparations have been used for centuries, and some dermatologists still employ sulphur ointment because it is inexpensive, safe, and effective. Benzyl benzoate was first used extensively in scabies treatment in 1937, and was the mainstay of therapy for many years. It is an extremely effective scabicide, but has irritant properties, and irritancy can be troublesome if the preparation is misused. γ-Benzene hexachloride (lindane) is also an effective scabicide, although there is now anecdotal evidence of lindane-resistant scabies in several parts of the world. A number of reports of neurotoxicity, usually in the form of seizures, has led to concern about the use of lindane, particularly in small children. However, in the majority of reported cases of neurotoxicity lindane had been misused or accidentally ingested. Malathion 0.5% in an aqueous base, marketed in the UK as Derbac-M liquid, does not appear to be as effective as benzylbenzoate or lindane in the treatment of scabies, and at least two separate applications are usually required to eliminate the infection. Monosulfiram (Tetmosol), although apparently not a widely used scabicide, is safe and effective. Monosulfiram containing soap has been used as a prophylactic measure in communities in which scabies is endemic.

A recent addition to the therapeutic armamentarium against scabies in the UK is 5% permethrin cream (Lyclear Dermal Cream). This preparation has been available in the USA for some time (Elimite), and appears to be a very effective scabicide. Lyclear Dermal Cream has a vanishing cream base, and one application, washed off after 8–24 h, should be effective in the majority of cases.

Hopefully, the presently available synthetic pyrethroids are the vanguard of many similar, 'environmentally friendly' pediculicides and acaricides.

Institutional outbreaks of scabies

There appears to have been a significant increase in the number of outbreaks of scabies in residential homes for the elderly in recent years. The dermatological literature contains numerous reports of scabies outbreaks in hospital wards and in residential homes, and in many of these reports the source of the infection was traced to a patient suffering from crusted (Norwegian) scabies. However, from personal experience of several of these outbreaks in residential homes for the elderly, I consider that it is more likely that the index case is a resident who is heavily infected, i.e. has a large parasite load, but who does not have classical crusted scabies. Such a patient will have large numbers of burrows on the hands and feet, and probably also on the trunk. They will therefore have an enormous number of mites in various stages of development on the skin surface. Some of these will be shed into the environment, and they will also be transmitted to nursing staff who come into contact with the patient. Nursing the elderly, who are frequently immobile, involves a great deal of physical contact between patient and nurse, and this facilitates transmission of mites. Nurses will often hold hands with elderly patients, either to steady them while they are walking, or simply as a gesture of affection or concern. If the nursing staff become infected, they may then spread the infection to other patients, and also to members of their own families.

It is obvious from this scenario that attempted eradication of an outbreak must involve treatment of every resident, every member of the nursing staff, and the members of the nurses' families. If, for example, only the residents are treated, then there is the possibility that they may be reinfected by nurses. The dermatologist must examine all residents in an attempt to identify the index case. Heavily infected patients will often require several treatments with a scabicide to eradicate their disease. All other residents should be treated on two occasions with a scabicide. There should be an interval of a few days between treatments. It is advisable for nursing staff and their families to follow the same regimen. Residents and nursing staff should then be examined 2–3 weeks after treatment to establish if there are any residual problems. If there is evidence of persisting infection then the treatment schedule should be repeated. If this routine is not adhered to, it is likely that the problem will persist.

The choice of scabicide is important. Many elderly patients with scabies have significant secondary eczematization, and benzylbenzoate will exacerbate this. The usual three-application schedule of benzylbenzoate treatment is also very time-consuming for nursing staff, particularly when large numbers of residents are to be treated. Derbac-M liquid is non-irritant, and easy to apply, but from personal experience I do not consider it to be as effective as some of the other scabicides. Lindane has proved very useful in this type of outbreak in the past but, as mentioned previously, there is increasing anecdotal evidence of the development of lindane-resistant scabies. I now consider that the most suitable preparation is Lyclear Dermal Cream.

Ordinary laundering of bed linen is sufficient to destroy the parasites. As an additional measure, carpets and soft furnishings in communal areas can be treated with an acaricide, and the local Environmental Health Department will advise on this.

Further reading

1 **Taplin D, Meinking TL,** Pyrethrins and pyrethroids in dermatology, *Arch Dermatol* (1990) **126**: 213–21.

2 **Burns DA,** The treatment of human ectoparasite infection, *Br J Dermatol* (1991) **125**: 89–93.

3 **Burns DA,** The treatment of *Pthirus pubis* infestation of the eyelashes, *Br J Dermatol* (1987) **117**: 741–3.

4 **Burns DA,** Diseases caused by arthropods and other noxious animals. In: Champion RH, Burton JL, Ebling FJG (eds). *Textbook of Dermatology*, 5th edn, Oxford: Blackwell Scientific, 1992, pp. 1265–324.

9

New indications for topical retinoids

Ronald Marks

Introduction

Since World War II there have been successive therapeutic 'waves,' each having its own dramatic effect but overall completely changing the face of dermatology. The introduction of the analogues of vitamin A (the retinoids) was one such wave.

Following anecdotal clinical reports of the efficacy of vitamin A itself in disorders as diverse as acne, psoriasis and pityriasis rubra pilaris, researchers investigated the effects of topical preparations of retinol and its esters. In the 1960s reports began to appear of the efficacy of the carboxylic acid of retinol (all-*trans*-retinoic acid (tretinoin)) and in 1971 topical tretinoin was introduced into the dermatological marketplace for the treatment of acne. Acne and other disorders characterized by follicular obstruction must be considered the 'classical use' of topical retinoids, and other topical retinoids, such as Motretinide, isotretinoin and CD271,

have been introduced for the same clinical purpose.

However, it has been clear since the first studies with topical tretinoin that there are several other potential therapeutic uses for this agent, and in the following some of these uses are highlighted.

Psoriasis

The comedolytic activity of topical tretinoin prompted investigators to examine the effects of the drug in other disorders characterized by the 'overproduction' of horn, including psoriasis. The initial report in 1969 of the effects of topical tretinoin in psoriasis[1] did indicate that there might be some therapeutic activity, but the effects seen in that study were not dramatic. Other reports of the action of topical tretinoin in psoriasis followed,[2–4] as did a study of the efficacy of the *cis* isomer, isotretinoin in this disease.[5] Curiously, however, it is only recently that the pharmaceutical industry has initiated detailed studies of a topical retinoid drug for the treatment of psoriasis. The agent concerned, AGN 190168, is an acetylenic retinoid, and initial studies indicate that it has useful therapeutic activity in plaque-type psoriasis. It is sad that, despite the fact that the potential therapeutic activity of a topical retinoid in psoriasis has been in the public arena for nearly 24 years, it is only recently that any real prospect of this potential being realized has emerged.

Table 9.1 Multicentre open study of 0.05% tretinoin cream in patients with solar keratoses*

	6 months *(n = 93)*		*9 months* *(n = 88)*		*12 months* *(n = 25)*		*15 months* *(n = 24)*	
	Pre	*Post*	*Pre*	*Post*	*Pre*	*Post*	*Pre*	*Post*
	11.2	8.9	11.2	7.9	14.4	8.84	14.0	7.4
Difference	2.2		3.4		5.5		6.6	
p	0.001		≤0.001		0.003		0.001	

Mean number of lesions before and after treatment (spanning header above)

Mean lesion size (mm²) before and after treatment

	6 months		*9 months*		*12 months*		*15 months*	
	Pre	*Post*	*Pre*	*Post*	*Pre*	*Post*	*Pre*	*Post*
	84.1	62.2	84.7	55.4	131.7	72.8	124.1	61.4
Difference	21.9		29.3		58.9		62.7	
p	0.001		≤0.001		0.014		0.009	

*Adapted from Kligman and Thorne.[9]

Non-melanoma skin cancer

One of the most exciting facts about the retinoids is that in some instances they are able to 'redirect' the abnormal differentiation of neoplastic tissue along more normal pathways. Inhibition of tumour progression by retinoid agents (chemoprevention rather than chemotherapy) has been reported in various animal models as well as in human disease.[6] This is certainly the case with premalignant epidermal lesions, as was first noticed by Stuttgen[7] more than 30 years ago with solar keratoses. In another study, Bollag and Ott[8] found that in 60 patients with solar keratoses treated with 0.1–0.3% topical tretinoin, 55% of those with facial lesions showed complete remission after 1–3 weeks and 39% showed a partial response to the treatment.

A much larger and more recent series of multicentre studies confirms

Table 9.2 Clinical response (%) obtained in multicentre, double-blind, vehicle-controlled studies of 6 months' treatment with 0.05% and 0.1% tretinoin cream

	0.05% cream	Vehicle	0.1% cream	Vehicle
Excellent	12.4	9.2	36.0	16.0
Good	29.2	24.6	37.0	24.0
Fair	34.4	25.0	15.0	24.0
Poor	24.0	24.0	12.0	35.0

*Adapted from Kligman and Thorne.[9]

the efficacy of treatment with 0.05% and 0.1% topical tretinoin creams.[9] The results of one of these studies are given in Table 9.1. Table 9.2 combines the results of two double-blind, vehicle-controlled studies lasting 6 months each. These studies indicate that topical tretinoin has a useful therapeutic effect in solar keratoses, and it is my belief that this agent is one important component of a regimen for patients with many such lesions and severe chronic photodamage.

Chronic photodamage

Apart from epidermal dysplasia and solar keratoses, individuals who have sustained a significant degree of solar damage develop a whole range of other lesions (Fig. 9.1). These are the result of solar elastotic degenerative change in dermal connective tissue and focal irregular disordered melanocytic activity. Fine lines around the mouth and eyes and deeper furrows at some exposed sites, a sallow yellowish discolouration, telangiectasia and purpura and lentigines are some of the sequelae of long continued exposure to the sun. These changes signify deranged skin function and are cosmetically displeasing. It was Albert Kligman[10] who first noticed that topical tretinoin could decrease the physical signs of photodamage. He observed that some of the older women with acne that he had been treating for long periods with topical tretinoin looked much less sun battered. These anecdotal clinical observations were followed by double-blind, vehicle-controlled studies which demonstrated beyond reasonable doubt that topical tretinoin had a striking therapeutic effect on photodamaged skin.[11–13] It became clear that the improvement was slow to develop, increased for periods of up to 1 year, and gradually relapsed when treatment stopped. Fine lines gradually decreased, and the sallowness so typical of solar elastosis diminished, being replaced by a 'rosy glow'. Telangiectasia became less prominent and the 'dyspigmentation' of solar damage, including solar lentigines, were found to fade in one study and became fewer in number after using

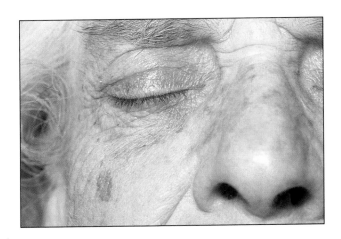

Figure 9.1

Photodamage of the upper part of the face showing many lines and sallow, yellowish discoloration and scattered brown marks (solar lintigines).

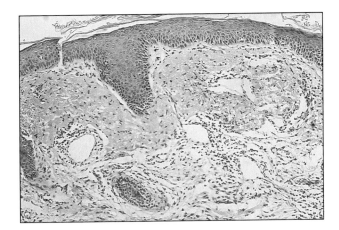

Figure 9.2

The histopathology of erythemato-telagiectic rosacea.

0.1% tretinoin cream for a 10-month period.[14]

Topical isotretinoin (0.05–0.1%) is also effective in chronic photodamage. Cunningham and his colleagues reported the results of a multicentre, randomized, vehicle-controlled, double-blind study in which 776 subjects were enrolled.[15] The subjects used 0.05% isotretinoin for 12 weeks and 0.1% for a further 24 weeks, or the vehicle for 36 weeks. The subjects were evaluated clinically using visual analogue scales and significant differences were found

($p<0.05$) at 36 weeks for overall skin appearance, fine wrinkles, sallowness and skin texture.

Many studies have also used objective techniques to record the improvement in physical signs. Optical profilometry in which image analysis is performed on standardized skin surface replicas before and after treatment with topical tretinoin has been one such successful approach.[16] Pulsed A-scan ultrasound has also been used in studies with topical tretinoin with skin thickening paralleling the clinical effects.[12,17] Objective 'blind' evaluation of clinical photographs has also been successfully employed to demonstrate the therapeutic effects of topical isotretinoin.[18]

The way(s) in which the topical retinoids work in chronic photodamage are not completely characterized. Epidermal thickening subsequent to increased mitotic activity is a well-known consequence of the application of topical retinoids.[19,20] New dermal blood vessel formation has been claimed after treatment with topical tretinoin for long periods and some work from the Cardiff group in which tissue Von Willebrand factor antigen was found to be increased after treatment of skin with topical tretinoin gives some support to this.[21] From studies in mice,[22,23] it would seem likely that new dermal connective tissue is synthesized and deposited subepidermally after treatment with topical retinoids, but this has not yet been satisfactorily demonstrated in human skin.

Regardless of how the topical retinoids exert their effects in chronic photodamage, there can be little doubt as to their efficacy and usefulness for this indication.

Rosacea

There is evidence that chronic photodamage is responsible for at least some of the signs and symptoms of rosacea.[24] In particular, the persistent erythema and telangiectasia may well be due to climatically damaged dermal connective tissue (Fig. 9.2). Kligman has recently reported that rosacea is improved by topical tretinoin in the long term,[24] and my own experience tends to confirm this. Clearly the action of topical retinoids in this disease may differ fundamentally from that of tetracycline or metronidazole, and many months may elapse before any improvement is recorded. However, it may well be that this approach is more successful for the erythema and telangiectasia than any of the other treatments available.

Conclusion

Topical retinoids were introduced more than 20 years ago but we are only now learning their full potential. As new topical retinoids with slightly different pharmacological and pharmaceutical profiles become available, it will be fascinating to find yet other therapeutic targets for their manifold actions.

References

1 Frost PH, Weinstein GD, Topical administration of vitamin A acid for ichthyosiform dermatoses and psoriasis, *JAMA* (1969) **207**: 1863–8.

2 Fredriksson T, Antipsoriatic activity of retinoic acid vitamin A acid, *Dermatologica* (1971) **142**: 133–6.

3 Fry L, MacDonald A, McMinn RMH, Effect of retinoic acid in psoriasis, *Br J Dermatol* (1970) **83**: 391–6.

4 Günther S, The therapeutic value of retinoic acid in chronic discoid, acute guttate and erythrodermic psoriasis: clinical observations on twenty-five patients, *Br J Dermatol* (1973) **89**: 515–7.

5 Bischoff R, de Jong EMGJ, Rulo HFC et al, Topical application of 13-cis-retinoic acid in the treatment of chronic plaque psoriasis, *Clin Exp Dermatol* (1992) **17**: 9–12.

6 Bollag W, Therapeutic effects of an aromatic retinoic acid analogue on chemically induced skin papilloma and carcinomas of mice, *Eur J Cancer* (1974) **10**: 731–7.

7 Stuttgen G, Zur Lokalbehandlung der Keratosen mit Vitamin A-Saure, *Dermatologica* (1962) **124**: 65–80.

8 Bollag W, Ott F, Retinoic acid: topical treatment of senile or actinic keratoses and basal cell carcinomas, *Agents Actions* (1970) **1**: 172–5.

9 Kligman AM, Thorne EG, Topical therapy of actinic keratoses with tretinoin, In: Marks R (ed). *Retinoids in cutaneous malignancy*, Oxford: Blackwell, 1991, pp. 66–73.

10 Kligman AM, Grove GL, Hirose R et al, Topical tretinoin for photoaged skin, *J Am Acad Dermatol* (1986) **15**: 836–59.

11 Ellis CN, Weiss JS, Hamilton TA et al, Sustained improvement with prolonged topical tretinoin (retinoic acid) for photoaged skin, *J Am Acad Dermatol* (1990) **23**: 629–37.

12 Lever L, Kumar P, Marks R, Topical retinoic acid for treatment of solar damage, *Br J Dermatol* (1990) **122**: 91–8.

13 Leyden JJ, Grove GL, Grove MJ et al, Treatment of photodamaged facial skin with topical tretinoin, *J Am Acad Dermatol* (1989) **21**: 638–44.

14 Rafal ES, Griffiths CEM, Ditre CM et al, Topical tretinoin (retinoic acid) treatment for liver spots associated with photodamage, *New Eng J Med* (1992) **326**(6): 368–74.

15 Cunningham WJ, Bryce GF, Armstrong RB et al, Topical isotretinoin and photodamage. In: Saurat J-H (ed). *Retinoids: 10 years on*, Basel: Karger, 1991, pp. 182–90.

16 Grove GL, Grove MJ, Leyden JJ, Optical profilometry: an objective method for quantification of facial wrinkles, *J Am Acad Dermatol* (1989) **21**: 631–7.

17 Marks R, Hill S, Barton SP, The effects of an abrasive agent on normal skin and on photoaged skin in comparison with topical tretinoin, *Br J Dermatol* (1990) **123**: 457–66.

18 Armstrong RB, Lesiewicz J, Harvey G et al, Clinical panel assessment of photodamaged skin treated with isotretinoin using photographs, *Arch Dermatol* (1992) **128**: 352–6.

19 Marks R, Pearse AD, Black D, Hill S, Techniques for assessing the activity of topically applied retinoids, *J Am Acad Dermatol* (1986) **15**(2): 810–6.

20 Lützow-Holm C, De Angelis P, Clausen OPF, Retinoic acid provokes a regeneration-like proliferative response in murine epidermis, *Arch Dermatol Res* (1992) **284**: 418–23.

21 Mourad MM, Marks R, Giddings J, Effects of retinoic acid and corticosteroids on capillary endothelium of human skin, *J Invest Dermatol* (1989) **92**(3), 393 (Abstr.).

22 Kligman LH, Duo CH, Kligman AM, Topical retinoic acid enhances the repair of ultraviolet-damaged dermal connective tissue, *Connective Tissue Res* (1984) **12**: 139–50.

23 Bryce GF, Bogdan NJ, Brown CC, Retinoic acids promote the repair of the dermal damage and the effacement of wrinkles in the UVB-irradiated hairless mouse, *J Invest Dermatol* (1988) **91**: 175–80.

24 Kligman AM, Topical tretinoin for rosacea: a preliminary report, *J Dermatol Treatment* (1993) **4**(2): 71–4.

10

New lamps for psoralen photochemotherapy of psoriasis

Peter M. Farr

Introduction

Since its introduction in the 1970s,[1] psoralen ultraviolet photochemotherapy (PUVA) has become a widely used second-line form of treatment for psoriasis. Although several therapeutic regimens have been described which differ with regard to the frequency of treatment and exposure doses used,[2-4] unlike ultraviolet B (UVB) phototherapy of psoriasis,[5] little attention has been paid to the light sources used in PUVA treatment. Lamps used for PUVA are almost invariably ultraviolet A (UVA) fluorescent lamps (such as the Philips TL09) with a fluorescence spectrum extending from around 320 to 400 nm, with a peak at 352 nm (Fig. 10.1).[6] The choice of this spectral power distribution was not made on the basis of therapeutic efficiency, but because these were the only lamps widely available when PUVA was introduced.

The therapeutic action spectrum (or wavelength dependence of therapeutic effect) for PUVA has been little studied. Psoralen–UVA erythema is the main limiting factor with regard to the dose of radiation that can be given at each treatment,[4] and action spectrum studies have shown that 8-methoxypsoralen applied topically increases the erythemal sensitivity of the skin from about 315 to 380 nm, with an apparent peak of photosensitivity at 330 nm.[7] By using equal erythemally effective doses of radiation from different light sources and observing the therapeutic response, it should be possible to determine whether the action spectra for psoralen erythema and the therapeutic effect diverge. If this is the case, then it should be possible to dissociate the erythemal response and therapeutic effect of PUVA and thus improve the effectiveness of treatment.

In this chapter two studies are reviewed in which the response of psoriasis to PUVA using different wavelengths was compared, and evidence is presented that UVB radiation may be effective in psoralen photochemotherapy.

UVA wavelength dependence in psoralen photochemotherapy

Brucke et al[8] studied three patients with chronic plaque type psoriasis using an irradiation monochromator

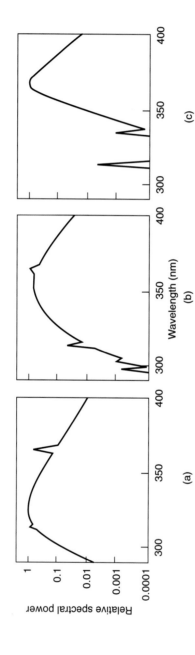

Figure 10.1

The spectral power distributions of the three ultraviolet fluorescent lamps used by Farr et al.[9] (a) 325 nm lamp; (b) 352 nm lamp (conventional PUVA lamp); (c) 370 nm lamp.

Table 10.1   The odds ratios for comparison of treatment with any two of the three lamps*

Lamps compared	Odds of shorter time to clearance with lamp listed second	95% confidence interval
370 nm vs. 352 nm	0.74	0.17, 3.57
352 nm vs. 325 nm	10.4	1.06, 102.1
370 nm vs. 325 nm	8.2	0.97, 69.5

*From Farr et al.[9]

set at a central wavelength of either 365±10 or 335±10 nm. The 72 h minimum phototoxic dose for each wavelength was determined by exposing four sites on uninvolved skin to increasing doses of radiation 1 h after ingestion of a liquid preparation of 8-methoxypsoralen, given at a standard dose of 0.6 mg/kg. Treatment was given four times weekly by exposing two 10 cm² sites within plaques of psoriasis using the previously determined minimal phototoxic dose at 365 or 335 nm. Subsequent dose increments were based on the clinical response.

The treated areas of psoriasis cleared completely in all three patients, irrespective of whether 335 or 365 nm radiation was used. Any difference in the rate of clearance for the two wavelengths was not discussed. The cumulative doses required for clearance were around 50% less at 335 nm compared with 365 nm, but this reduction was in proportion to the difference in minimum phototoxic doses at the two wavelengths. Thus the conclusion from this study was that 365 and 335 nm radiation, when given in equal erythemal doses, had an equal therapeutic effect and that there was no evidence to suggest that the action spectra for psoralen erythema and clearance of psoriasis were dissociated.

Farr et al,[9] rather than using an irradiation monochromator to study a small area of psoriasis, used three different types of UVA fluorescent lamp allowing exposure of a larger area of skin. The lamps had peak emission at 325, 352 (the conventional PUVA lamp) or 370 nm (Fig. 10.1). Fifteen of each of the lamps were mounted in a cylindrical configuration to allow exposure of the whole of a patient's forearm. A total of 24 patients were studied, each with psoriasis affecting both forearms to approx-

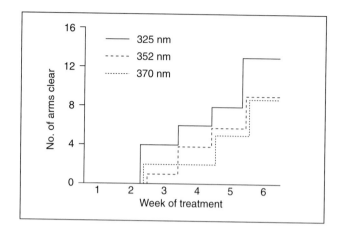

Figure 10.2

Clearance of psoriasis according to week of treatment with each of the three lamps.

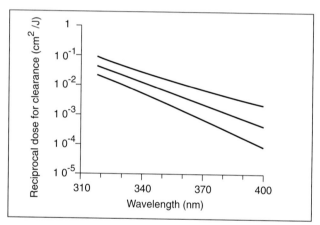

Figure 10.3

Exponential action spectrum and 95% confidence limits for the clearance of psoriasis by oral 80-methoxypsoralen photochemotherapy. (From Farr et al.[9])

imately the same severity and extent. The patients were allocated randomly to be treated with two of the fluorescent lamp units (one for each arm). Treatment, 2 h after ingestion of crystalline 8-methoxypsoralen at a standard dose of 0.6 mg/kg, was given three times weekly for 6 weeks, with the starting dose based on 40% of the minimum phototoxic dose, calculated for the appropriate lamps in each patient. Doses were increased by 40% after each block of three treatments, unless burning occurred. Assessment of response was made by one clinician who was unaware of the types of lamps being used in individual patients, and who made a simple comparison between the two arms in each patient.

Arms treated with the 325 nm lamps were found to clear with significantly fewer treatments than with the other two lamp types (Table 10.1, Fig. 10.2), but without increased risk of burning. These results suggest that erythema and therapeutic effect in PUVA treatment can be dissociated at shorter wavelengths (325 nm) than those used conventionally (352 nm).

Based on the doses of radiation required for clearance of psoriasis with each of the lamp types, Farr et al[9] proposed an action spectrum for the clearance of psoriasis by psoralen photochemotherapy using an exponential function which suggested that radiation at 320 nm was an order of magnitude more effective than that at 360 nm (Fig. 10.3).

Response of psoriasis to psoralen UVB photochemotherapy

A narrow-band UVB fluorescent lamp (Philips TL01) with 83% of its ultraviolet emission at 311 ± 2 nm has been shown to be highly effective in the UVB phototherapy of psoriasis.[10] Sakuntabhai et al[11] have investigated the use of this lamp in psoralen photochemotherapy. Ten patients with psoriasis affecting both forearms to approximately the same severity and extent were studied. In each case, one forearm was allocated randomly to receive UVB therapy alone (0.7 J/cm²), and the other forearm to receive the same dose of radiation 2 h after ingestion of a standard dose of 8-methoxypsoralen (0.6 mg/kg). Treatment was given twice weekly until the lesions on one forearm had cleared.

In eight of the nine patients who completed the trial, the psoralen–UVB treated arm cleared before the UVB treated arm; clearance was equal in one patient (Fig. 10.4). Very few psoralen–UVB treatments (median number 5) were required for clearance of psoriasis and none of the patients developed painful erythema. This study has therefore established that psoralen–UVB therapy is more effective than UVB phototherapy alone. That this improved response was not accompanied by a greater incidence of erythema or other acute side-effects suggests that erythema and therapeutic effect may be dissociable. Clearly, further studies are required to establish whether psoralen–UVB therapy is more effective than conventional PUVA treatment.

Conclusions

The action spectrum for clearance of psoriasis with psoralen photochemotherapy has not yet been fully established, although there is strong evidence from one study that shorter wavelengths (around 325 nm) are more effective than wavelengths conventionally used for PUVA (352 nm), or longer wavelengths (370 nm). Unfortunately, the 325 nm lamps used

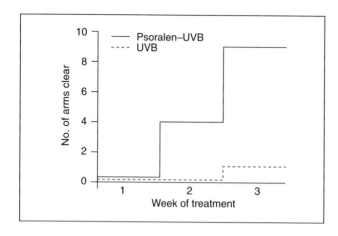

Figure 10.4

Clearance of psoriasis according to week of treatment with UVB or psoralen–UVB exposure.

by Farr et al[9] are no longer available and no similar fluorescent lamp is presently manufactured. Filtered metal halide lamps[5] are available for use in PUVA therapy as an alternative to fluorescent lamps. Although only used in approximately 4% of dermatology units in the UK,[6] they are apparently more popular in other European countries.[12] Metal halide lamps have a bias towards longer wavelengths when compared with conventional PUVA lamps and so, on the basis of the action spectrum presented in Fig. 10.3, are likely to be less effective.

The response of psoriasis to UVB photochemotherapy (using 311 nm lamps) is presently being further investigated. If a dissociation between erythema and therapeutic effect is confirmed in studies of whole-body treatment, then psoralen photochemotherapy using 311 nm lamps (PUVB) may be expected to have less short-term

risks than conventional PUVA. As 311 nm lamps are also effective in the treatment of psoriasis with ultraviolet radiation alone, psoralen photochemotherapy or ultraviolet phototherapy could be performed with the same lamp, avoiding duplication of irradiation equipment.

References

1 Parrish JA, Fitzpatrick TB, Tanenbaum L et al, Photochemotherapy of psoriasis with oral methoxalen and long wave ultraviolet light, *N Engl J Med* (1974) **291**: 1207–11.

2 Melski JW, Tanenbaum L, Parrish JA et al, Oral methoxalen photochemotherapy for the treatment of psoriasis: a cooperative clinical trial, *J Invest Dermatol* (1977) **68**: 328–35.

3 Henseler T, Wolff K, Honigsmann H et al, Oral 8-methoxypsoralen photochemotherapy of psoriasis. The

European PUVA study: a cooperative study among 18 European centres, *Lancet* (1981) **i**: 853–7.

4 **Sakuntabhai A, Sharpe GR, Farr PM,** Response of psoriasis to twice weekly PUVA, *Br J Dermatol* (1993) **128**: 166–71.

5 **Diffey BL, Farr PM,** An appraisal of ultraviolet lamps used for the phototherapy of psoriasis, *Br J Dermatol* (1987) **117**: 49–56.

6 **Farr PM, Diffey BL,** PUVA treatment of psoriasis in the United Kingdom, *Br J Dermatol* (1991) **124**: 365–7.

7 **Cripps DJ, Lowe NJ, Lerner AB,** Action spectra of topical psoralens: a re-evaluation, *Br J Dermatol* (1982) **107**: 77–82.

8 **Brucke J, Tanew A, Ortel B et al,** Relative efficacy of 335 and 365 nm radia-tion in photochemotherapy of psoriasis, *Br J Dermatol* (1991) **124**: 372–4.

9 **Farr PM, Diffey BL, Higgins EM et al,** The action spectrum between 320 and 400 nm for clearance of psoriasis by psoralen photochemotherapy, *Br J Dermatol* (1991) **124**: 443–8.

10 **van Weelden H, Baart de la Faille H, Young E et al,** A new development in UVB phototherapy of psoriasis, *Br J Dermatol* (1988) **119**: 11–19.

11 **Sakuntabhai A, Diffey BL, Farr PM,** Response of psoriasis to psoralen-UVB photochemotherapy, *Br J Dermatol* (1993) **128**: 296–300.

12 **Calzavara-Pinton PG, Rastrelli M, Carlino A et al,** PUVA treatment of psoriasis in Italy, *Br J Dermatol* (1992) **127**: 548.

11

Principles, practice and ethics of clinical trials

Medical ethics—the doctor's view

Stephen E. Smith

As a physician from a totally different discipline, it is very flattering to be invited to contribute to this text on dermatological treatments. I have had only a little dermatological experience, but as House Physician at St Thomas's Hospital in the early 1950s I was obliged to clerk many severely eczematous patients under the care of Dr Geoffrey Dowling and to carry out his orders for their treatment. It was a time when systemic corticosteroid therapy was being introduced and its dangers were already perceived, but topical cortisone had already been observed to fail, presumably because it did not penetrate the skin. At the time, treatment had not advanced far beyond that available in the previous decade and it included vitamin supplements, ergosterol, topically applied tomato leaves, intravenous procaine, intradermal serum, alcohol injection and many others. The one I administered and recall most vividly, because it was so dramatic, was intravenous typhoid/paratyphoid A and B vaccine (TAB).

With what glee we stood at the end of the bed an hour later to witness the unfortunate patient's rigor, sure in our belief that this onslaught would do him or her some good.

Such reminiscences by the elderly are apt to focus a reader's attention in particular on the writer's age, but in this instance I hope a point can be made. Some of these patients undoubtedly improved; they spent a while in hospital and that may have helped, or indeed the shock therapy may have activated the pituitary– adrenal axis sufficiently to ameliorate their condition. Referring to non-specific protein therapy in dermatology, Bray[1] expressed the opinion that none had any special virtue and that 'the injection may keep a patient interested whilst Nature cures him'. I have subsequently scoured the literature back to the early years of this century and can find no published evidence of a controlled trial of this type of treatment. Such a trial should indeed have been performed because, apart from doubts about its efficacy and the unpleasantness of the febrile reaction produced, intravenous TAB was already known to cause haemorrhagic reactions and neurotoxicity.

There was a need to know. Patients should have been brought into hospital (I do not recall a bed shortage in those days; if an extra one was needed you put it up in the middle of the ward) and entered into a randomized double-blind placebo-controlled parallel group clinical trial and the bona fide effects of the treatment assessed with rating scales of subjective symptoms and records of skin area and thickness, temperature, cellularity and time to resolution (if any).

In a later age there would have been another 'need to know'—How does the treatment work, and if we knew that would it help us to understand better the nature of the condition being treated? Let us take small skin biopsies before, during and after treatment to explore their microscopic appearance and the chemical behaviour of their cells, receptors and messengers. Furthermore, to define more precisely the disease and its response to medication, let us do parallel experiments on healthy volunteers. In a still later age when monetary contraints assail us, there is a further 'need to know', at the present time a crucial one. How much does it cost, how long will the patient be in hospital, can it be done as an outpatient, will the GP pay for it? and so on. The questions at every age are endless and everyone, patient, doctor, nurse, paramedic, administrator, finance director and politician alike, wants to know the answers.

There was once a time when everyone trusted the medical practitioner to do all that was necessary, to administer the best treatment, to find the answers to important questions without harming anyone, to be kind, thoughtful and honest, and never to betray that trust. It is customary to attribute the present downturn to the appalling activities of the Nazi doctors who betrayed humanity at the behest of their ideological masters. In fact, the betrayal in a less dramatic way, began much earlier. One has only to search the literature of the 18th century (Smollett had much to say on the subject) to realize that many doctors were dishonest and covered up their ignorance and their errors of omission and commission to the detriment of their patients. In our own era medical misbehaviour unfortunately did not end with the Nazis and there are innumerable published examples of research in which abuse of patients is all too prominent. Those who doubt should read Pappworth's passionate indictment, published in 1967,[2] or recall the episodes involving children at the Willowbrook school or patients in the town of Tuskegee, Alabama.

For these and other reasons, Society now understandably demands that all research on man be subject to review by duly appointed Ethics Committees. Such Committees are charged with assessing the rightness or wrongness of such research and of granting or withholding approval for investigations to go ahead. My only personal qualification for standing before you today is that I have been Chairman of one such Ethics Committee for the past 9 years and have thereby a wealth of experience on which to draw. That experience is restricted to the ethics of research and I shall therefore confine this talk to that area. I must point out that I am not a trained ethicist (whatever such an animal may be) and certainly not a trained lawyer. My philosophy for experimentation is strictly a personal one founded on a Christian and humanitarian tradition and strongly influenced by perceptions of the dictates of good science as well as the needs of Society. I am a passionate believer in the National Health Service and through it in the rights of individuals to obtain the best medical care. In my years as a Chairman I have been warmly supported, greatly helped and well guided by many people. In the dermatological field I would like to pay tribute in particular to Professors Robin Eady and Richard Camp, whose expertise and advice have been invaluable. I should perhaps explain that we have one consultant member from the Institute of Dermatology by right. I have been fortunate also in having a devoted lay membership from which I continue to learn on every occasion that we meet.

Ethics Committees up and down the country are composed largely of willing but untrained people such as myself. Fortunately, many sources of guidance are available to us: those of the World Medical Association (formulated in the Declaration of Helsinki), directives of the Medical Research Council and the Association of the British Pharmaceutical Industry, by the Royal College of Physicians and by many distinguished individuals such as McCance, Bradford Hill and Fox and by Pope Pius XII. The moral and ethical perceptions of these individuals and groups are similar. Because the available literature is so enriched by the wisdom contained within these sources, I shall not try to improve upon it, but rather to select a number of ethical problems, old and new, which appear to me to merit close attention.

Whether we signed the oath or not, every one of us operates in accordance with the Hippocratic principle which states that a prime responsibility of the doctor lies in the safeguarding of the health of his or her patients. At first sight simple, the principle is not always easy to follow in research practice. There are, for example, clinical-trial situations in which it is necessary to stop a regular treatment in order to test a new one satisfactorily. It could be risky or at least disadvantageous to the individual patient, though the information gained from a trial in which this was done might be important to medical science and could be beneficial to other patients in the future. The situation is one of conflict between the needs of the individual and those of Society; it requires careful examination of the scale and nature of both the risks and the likely benefits.

Another principle is less contentious. It is that if a new untried aid to diagnosis or treatment offers real hope to patients then the doctor must be free to use it. In such circumstances, I hold that forced reference to a Committee implies forced delegation of professional responsibility. Wherever possible, we have always refused to condone the practice and that for the most part is the accepted norm in this country. In the USA, however, this is not so and I have received many requests to authorize the provision of new drugs on a named-patient basis. The demands are usually placed by pharmaceutical companies who, though willing to offer help, try to avoid the risk of litigation should something go wrong. In this context I find that doctors need to be reminded that in their treatment of individual patients they are in law free to use any method and are certainly not bound by the indications for use set out in the Medicinal Product Licence. If you chose to treat warts by application of sulphuric acid, that is a matter for professional judgement; it is not illegal.

For the most part, we take the general view that the Committee's approval is required only for research. Where a study is done primarily for the benefit of the patient we do not need to be involved, and if a study is being done both for the benefit of the patient and for research purposes, then the investigator must try and assess which comes first. It is not always easy and one recognizes a kind of grey area in which we make the decision which seems best at the time. What is of course certain is that the needs of science and of Society, certainly those of the pharmaceutical industry, must never take precedence over considerations related to the well-being of the subject.

I come now to the cornerstone of my chapter. It is that to be ethical research must be scientifically valid. From this it follows that the most minor procedure such as the taking of a single blood sample or even administration of a questionnaire may be unethical if there is insufficient scientific basis. We recently turned down a proposal to measure plasma cortisol in a study of pituitary–adrenal suppression in children receiving inhaled corticosteroids; the investigators had already told us that their primary measure of suppression was the level of 24 h urinary endogenous steroid output. We concluded that inadequate reason existed for venepuncture. By contrast, a major procedure such as insertion of a cardiac catheter or the taking of a biopsy may be ethical, always provided that there is adequate scientific justification.

The matter would seem so obvious as to need no statement, yet we are presented with all too many proposals that are based on poor science and which have to go back and be replanned. Perhaps the two common-est faults are the following. The first is in the uncontrolled clinical trial in which a medicinal substance is given to patients without a parallel control group and without crossover, or perhaps with a parallel group treated with an inappropriate control medica-tion. Pharmaceutical companies are the worst offenders. They are, or feel they are, under pressure to generate data, maybe for advertisements or brochures but often for licensing submissions, which are not subject to quite the same intense scrutiny as accompanies sub-mission to peer-reviewed journals. An author has recently castigated a number of journals for publishing symposia constructed of this kind of endeavour. I believe prospective inves-tigators should resist invitations to do this kind of research, however elegantly it is dressed up.

The second fault is exclusive to investigators. It arises from a failure to examine statistical aspects of their studies. Most often they plan to recruit too few patients and thereby deny themselves adequate power to detect a change of the size they seek. Many people find it hard to credit that you can actually calculate how many patients are needed for a clinical trial in a situation where you do not know how effective the drug will be. The answer of course is that one can never predict the effectiveness of a drug or treatment regime in advance, but what you can do is define what clinical effect would be worth having. If I go to Professor Cunliffe with a new agent for reducing the number of spots on teenagers' faces, what I shall ask him is what size of reduction is clinically worthwhile; perhaps he will say 50%. I do not know. If one can answer these questions, finding the numbers is easy. If one cannot answer them, then the research may not be worth doing and if it is done with inadequate numbers then it will be unethical because the true expectation is of no decisive or useful outcome. I was recently forced to advise one group of investigators that a particular question they wanted to address within their unit could be answered only with a very large-scale multicentre trial.

In the context of scientific justifica-tion, I would like to consider now two matters which I think affect all research. The first is concerned with what at first sight appears an obvious question—Has this research been done before and, if so, is there already a clear answer to the problem which is to be addressed? It is rightly accepted practice that if you do not know what has already been done then you conduct a literature search to find out. Then you make a decision about whether or not to proceed according to the published observations. It could reasonably be held that to repeat any piece of research, if the answer is already known, is unethical because the risk–benefit equation is now grossly distorted. But the issues are not inevitably clear-cut. First, CD-ROM searches do not always yield all one is looking for; it takes persistence and often ingenuity, and one may miss something. Comfortingly, there are now moves to establish a registration system so that all clinical trials will be subject to recall.[3] Secondly, and more crucially, however, supposing the research has been done before but the confidence intervals of the outcome were not sufficiently confined to persuade doctors to act on that outcome, it might then be ethical to repeat the experiment. But how many times could one legitimately go on doing so again and again? At some stage, or perhaps at every stage, someone has to evaluate all the research by performance of a meta-analysis. Lau[4] has recently done sequential meta-analyses on all the published placebo-controlled trials of streptokinase after acute myocardial infarction. The results show clearly that the average outcome and acceptable confidence intervals could have been known in 1977. Yet it was after this date that the two most famous clinical trials,

ISIS-II and GISSI, which recruited huge numbers of patients, were performed. If one assumes that at that stage the profession had adopted streptokinase as part of routine management, as perhaps they should, then further confirmatory trials would surely have been unethical. A simple calculation, based on the numbers of patients who received injections of the placebo, shows that 500 fewer patients would have died as a result. I suppose it could be argued that it took two enormous trials to persuade the profession to adopt the treatment, but I suspect that the truth is that nobody troubled to look. In this instance I find ethics really rather difficult. As Rudolf Steiner once pointed out, there is a great difference between right and wrong, but sometimes it is difficult to tell which is which!

It could be held that, so long as valid informed consent is obtained from the participants, then any research will be ethical. The judges at the Nuremberg Military Tribunal rightly stipulated that 'The voluntary consent of the human subject is absolutely essential. This means that the person involved should have legal capacity to give consent; should be so situated as to be able to exercise free power of choice...'. We all agree with the premise, but unfortunately informed consent is incredibly difficult to define except in the broadest legal terms, one reason being that we can rarely agree on how much information is needed to make a valid judgement. Does one recruit black healthy volunteers to research involving the taking of skin biopsies, so long as they are informed that there is a risk of keloid formation involved? Does anyone know the odds? I suspect not. For the umpteenth trial of streptokinase, do you tell the subject all about the previous trials and the odds ratios already discovered? Will he understand what it really means?

I have reached an age of realization of how little I do understand, especially when registrars provide me with very careful guidance on some newly discovered matter of science. Further I have lost much of the capacity to understand that I once had. When the great Sydney Smith offered an explanation of some intricate matter of law to the bench and the judge said as a result that he was 'none the wiser', Smith is reputed to have remarked 'Maybe not, my Lord, but possibly better informed'. Most of our patients understand little of medical science and they know less. What then can one usefully tell them? The medical profession in this country still adopts a paternalistic attitude which many of us think suits us, though I am not sure that our patients agree. As a result we tend to produce information sheets or consent forms which have on them only that information which we believe the patient needs to know. By contrast, in the USA patients have absolute rights to know everything, and consequently their information sheets are very long and often indigestible. In my opinion it is counterproductive to give people too much data to assimilate

because of the indigestion which results, but I must admit that knowing just where to draw the line is sometimes difficult. I have always relied on the lay members in our Committee; they seem to be better at it than are the doctors.

Finally, I would like to touch on two ethical matters which we must address in the near future. When we do so, both will land us in conflict with our financial and political masters. The first relates to indemnity and compensation for injury. Many experimental studies and clinical trials are sponsored by pharmaceutical companies who carry indemnity and agree to abide by the ABPI guidelines for compensation. That is admirable. But we also do unsponsored studies and in most institutions those carry no insurance cover at all. The best hope for the individual who is injured as a result of taking part in such a study is that he will receive an ex gratia payment. Knowing the perilous state of many District Health Authorities and Trust finances, I consider that situation to be unacceptable. If the subject is a healthy volunteer who is not registered as a patient or client of the Authority then the situation could be even worse, for then there is no basis for a claim against the doctor or his employer on grounds of negligence except possibly in common law. I have already tried to get the situation changed, so far in vain, and I most earnestly urge you to do likewise.

The other problem for the future arises in the field of patient management. Doctors are now required to audit the things they do, so as to be able to provide answers to questions such as 'How effective is your management of patients and their conditions?', 'How much does it cost?' and 'What are the alternatives?'. I am all in favour. As a scientist, however, I want to make sure that if changes are introduced they are soundly based on good research and not on financial expediency or on political ideology. In recent years we have seen the closing of most psychiatric hospitals and the discharge of patients into the community. However well conceived this may have been, it was never subject to any proper research, the promised level of community support service has not appeared and, as a result, there are now more mentally ill people in prison than ever before and our large towns have within them cardboard cities of unprecedented size. My message here is: if administrators or others want to introduce changes in the way patients are managed, please try to ensure that it is done on the basis of properly conducted research. *Inter alia*, this will require establishment of the closest possible liaison between Ethics and Audit Committees and management themselves.

I started by referring to a piece of history, the use of intravenous TAB in the management of serious skin disease. Perhaps a word of reassurance is in order; I am not about to persuade my dermatological colleagues to do a clinical trial with it. What I am about to do, and what I have tried to do here, is to express my conviction that all research and evaluation of every kind should be soundly and scientifically based. In a section devoted to medical ethics, that is at least this doctor's view.

References

1 **Bray GW**, Non-specific protein therapy, *Practitioner* (1933) **130**: 545–63.

2 **Pappworth MH**, *Human guinea-pigs: experimentation in man*, London: Routledge & Kegan Paul, 1967.

3 **Chalmers I, Dickersin K, Chalmers TC et al**, Getting to grips with Archie Cochran's agenda. All randomised controlled trials should be registered and reported, *Br Med J* (1992) **305**: 786–7.

4 **Lau J, Anthian EM, Jiminez-Silva J et al**, Cumulative meta-analysis of therapeutic trials for myocardial infarction, *New Engl J Med* (1992) **327**: 248–54.

12

Statistical approaches to clinical trials

Colin B. Blakemore

Introduction

All of us are familiar with jocular (*sic*) references to 'lies, damned lies, and statistics', or even more pointedly to the fact that 'there are lies and there are damned lies, just as there are statistics and our statistics'. Such public disapproval pays tribute to an understanding that today many aspects of social policy and administration are determined by statistical considerations. To those of you involved in applied clinical research the value of a statistical approach to the organization and evaluation of data is widely accepted, and in no area more so than in the planning, design, and analysis of clinical trials. In this last statement I acknowledge the role of a statistical approach, and hence of the statistician, not only in the analysis and interpretation of data accumulated during clinical trials, but also an involvement in the earliest stages of research planning and trial design.

The importance of statistical input at the planning and trial design stage of clinical research cannot be overstressed, because whilst clinicians emphasize the importance of appropriate 'statistics' when discussing trial outcomes, many appear not to fully understand that the statistical analysis is usually predetermined by the design of the trial. Indeed, I would go so far as to suggest that unless a clinician has a sound grasp of mathematics together with some formal training in statistics, they would be well advised to treat the analysis of data as a statistician's 'black-box' activity; there are many excellent books written to help clinicians to understand, interpret, and evaluate the products of this black-box, of which I would strongly recommend the recent *New England Journal of Medicine* publication edited by Bailar and Mosteller.[1] The area in which a meaningful and valuable technical dialogue between clinician and statistician can occur, surrounds those questions of design and administration with which each planned clinical trial begins. In the remainder of this chapter, I intend to examine questions of trial design and administration as they apply to clinical research in dermatology.

Controlled vs open clinical trials

The preference for a controlled trial over an open study is undeniable when therapeutic efficacy is the primary aim of a trial, with the control against which the treatment under investigation is compared being either an existing proven therapy or a placebo. Only in an appropriately controlled trial can we draw statistically justifiable inferences, expressed as the probability of a chance finding, regarding the superiority of one treatment over another. All of this does not preclude an open trial from fulfilling a useful research role, generating data which can be statistically evaluated; instances which spring immediately to mind are those in which the primary aim of the trial is to evaluate the extent and width of a therapeutic window under different dosage regimens, or in which some attribute of the trial is to be evaluated, e.g. the irritancy of a transdermal delivery system patch. Before leaving the open, uncontrolled trial it should be emphasized that such trials are most likely to generate undisputed findings when patient stratification, either demographic or disease related, is built into the trial design or is defined and examined at the time of analysis of the data.

Having decided on the degree and type of controlled observations to be accumulated during the trial, we turn to the question of patient numbers. Together with the probability level at which we will reject findings as being due to chance, the size of the patient sample will ultimately determine the *power* of the statistical analysis, and hence the validity of inferences drawn from the trial data. The two principal errors we can make in the statistical analysis are: (a) to detect a significant difference between treatment effects when none exist in reality (type I error); and (b) to fail to detect a true difference in treatment effects (type II error). The power of the statistical analysis to avoid type I errors is dependent on the probability level at which we will treat findings as 'significant', while type II errors are dependent on the size of the trial sample. Establishing the optimal sample size for a clinical trial, to provide sufficient power to validate and justify the statistical findings, is a task best left to a statistician, who will know how to use correctly sets of tables specifically geared towards the design of clinical trials such as those produced by Machin and Campbell.[2] Another feature of clinical trial design which is influenced by the choice of sample size, is the use of non-parametric statistical procedures as opposed to parametric methods during the statistical analysis: irrespective of the type of measurements recorded to evaluate therapeutic response (continuous vs. discrete, quantitative vs. qualitative) unless the sample size is substantial, with values approximating a normal distribution, non-parametric procedures should always be preferred.

Controlled comparative trials

Controlled clinical trials all involve designs in which patients are treated with different therapies, one of which might be an inactive placebo, and the response to treatment is then compared. In the simplest of these designs patients are randomly allocated to different groups, each of which receives a different therapy. The statistical analysis of such trials is fairly straightforward, with appropriate non-parametric or parametric statistical procedures being applied to reveal differences in therapeutic response. Usually, this type of group comparative design involves 'repeated measures', in that each patient contributes a pretreatment and post-treatment assessment of disease severity, and perhaps also additional assessments during the course of treatment; because of these repeated measurements the statistical techniques employed during the analysis have to be appropriate to models in which both intraindividual changes and interindividual differences can be accommodated without distorting the differences between groups of patients on different treatments. Another source of difficulty which has to be taken into account during the analysis, and which must be addressed in the trial design, relates to the fact that it is frequently found that more than one measure of therapeutic response is incorporated into a trial. The occurrence of 'multiple end-points' in a trial, generates special problems for the analysis to ensure that significant findings which occur in the data have not happened by chance within the evaluation of a large number of end-

points, each of which has a specific probability of an erroneous significant finding occurring by chance alone. The way to avoid such complications, is to keep the number of end-points to as few as possible, and to ensure that each end-point is as precisely and distinctively defined as possible.

Patients as their own controls

Crossover clinical trials administer each treatment to each patient, so that the patient provides his own control: in a trial involving two treatments (known as a 'two-period crossover trial') each patient receives each treatment for a given period of time, usually with a washout period between treatments, with the order of treatments being randomized between patients. The statistical comparison of treatments (periods) in the crossover trial, is legitimate only if no carryover between periods is found, indicating that therapeutic response during the first period does not influence therapeutic response during the second period. If carryover is present then the statistical analysis has to be restricted to the comparison of first period treatments only, by which the trial has become a simple group comparative trial. One of the attractions of crossover designs is that sample sizes can be kept low because each patient contributes more than one therapeutic response. Unfortunately, in the majority of therapeutic response situations to demonstrate an absence of carryover requires substantial numbers of patients in each treatment period, and so the advantage of smaller sample sizes is lost; also it must be remembered that to have sufficient power for the statistical analysis to be valid, there must be sufficient patients on each treatment during the first period to support a comparative analysis. In recent years a number of valuable books have been published on crossover designs, of which those by Jones and Kenward[3] and Senn[4] are strongly recommended.

In dermatological clinical trials the classic crossover design is seldom employed, but a hybrid design which has many features in common with the crossover design is frequently employed to use the patient as his or her own control; this is the so called 'bilateral' design, in which sites of comparable disease severity on each side of the body simultaneously receive different therapies. There are many technical problems which make the statistical analysis of bilateral trial data complicated and prone to considerable error, primarily caused by the non-independence of observations of therapeutic response and the correlation of therapeutic outcomes: but the bilateral clinical trial can be analysed with acceptable levels of statistical power, and the patient does truly act as his own control. I must point out, however, that my experience in the analysis of such trials suggests that many dermatological trialists adopt a practice which is not appropriate, and which cannot be handled within a statistical analysis. The practice to which I refer is to treat the bilateral sites as if they represent therapeutic responses which are distinct and separated both spatially and temporally, and hence symptoms such as erythema, itch, etc., are assessed for each site and these responses are then statistically analysed as if drawn from different patients. Such practice generates data in which so much correlated error exists that formal statistical analysis of the data becomes a highly dubious exercise: of course the bilateral design can be used to *compare* the two sites, in terms such as 'equally improved', 'right better than left', 'no response in either site (side)', etc., and such assessments of therapeutic response can be analysed statistically with some very powerful procedures.

References

1 **Bailar JC, Mosteller F,** *Medical uses of statistics,* Boston: NEJM, 1992.

2 **Machin D, Campbell MJ,** *Statistical tables for the design of clinical trials,* Oxford: Blackwell, 1987.

3 **Jones B, Kenward MG,** *Design and analysis of cross-over trials,* London: Chapman & Hall, 1989.

4 **Senn S,** *Cross-over trials in clinical research,* Chichester: Wiley, 1993.

13

Clinical trials—methods of assessment

Ronald Marks

Introduction

The past 40 years has seen a revolution in the way that physicians decide on the most appropriate treatment for particular patients. No longer are pseudo-scientific rationalizations or folkloric explanations acceptable steps in the choice of a remedy. Quite understandably we are expected to know which is the most effective and least hazardous drug to use in a particular circumstance, and to defend the choice if challenged. One of the implications of medical audit may be that we are acting unprofessionally if we fail to pay attention to this expectation.

To live up to this ideal of knowing which is the most useful and least toxic remedy available there is a need to publish data from well-performed clinical trials, and this contribution to the symposium concerns the techniques that can be employed to monitor drug effects in these trials.

Why is measurement necessary?

Unfortunately, few drugs have the dramatic efficacy of penicillin, and in many instances their therapeutic effects are subtle and may be difficult to distinguish from those of a placebo. To reveal the small response from such medicaments a quantitative comparison of the rate of change in symptoms and/or signs with those of a control (usually placebo treated) group is needed. A further important use of measurement in the context of clinical trials is comparison between the different active treatments available in order to determine the rank order of their efficacies. Rank ordering toxicities as well as charting and comparing the time-course of any drug effects induced are other functions made possible by measurement. It should be possible to determine the exact rate of improvement with different treatments and this information, together with data on toxicity, bioavailability and cost, should remove some of the traditional guesswork from therapeutics.

If appropriate measures of disease phenomena are made during a clinical trial employing different drug doses, then it will also be possible to determine a dose–effect relationship. Knowledge of this allows estimation of the optimum dose and assessment of the dose at which no further benefit will occur, as well as the dose at which there is an increased likelihood of toxicity.

It is difficult to imagine a trial of a hypertensive agent without serial measures of blood pressure, or an assessment of an antidiabetic agent without measures of blood sugar. Surely dermatologists should subscribe to the same philosophy and those of us interested in therapy for skin disease should employ objective measures of skin disorder whenever possible.

Requirements of a measurement technique

No clinical measuring technique is perfect, but in the context of a dermatological clinical trial some characteristics are mandatory, some important and some highly desirable, and others useful and/or interesting but not vital.

Mandatory characteristics

Relevance and accuracy

It is essential that any technique for quantifying a clinical feature is relevant to assessment of progress of the disease in question. For example, there is no point in measuring the degree of scaling in acne because this clinical sign, if present in this disease, would have no relevance to the progress of the disorder being treated. Accuracy implies that the measurement taken is a truthful recording of the phenomenon targeted and, for example, a technique to measure the degree of scaling should measure this feature alone and not be contaminated by other features such as skin colour. Without assurance on both the relevance of a measurement and its accuracy, the measurement technique under discussion may supply data that are unreliable and difficult to interpret.

Reproducibility and repeatability

Repeatability signifies that the same answer is obtained when the measurement is repeated in the same circumstances. Reproducibility signifies that the same result is obtainable by another worker in another laboratory on another occasion who is trying to measure the same clinical phenomenon. Clearly it is vital that there are high levels of both repeatability and reproducibility. A coefficient of reproducibility of 5% or less is highly desirable, but regrettably not always obtained with current skin measuring devices. It must also be admitted that with some techniques (e.g. questionnaires assessing personality or disability, or measurements of skin extensibility), making the measurement itself alters the measurand, and this prevents accurate assessment of repeatability.

Sensitivity and linearity

It is essential that the technique used is sufficiently sensitive to record the smallest change likely to be induced by the therapeutic intervention being submitted to trial. Although the effect of a drug may not always produce a linear dose–effect response in the tissue being monitored it is vital that the parameter to be recorded has an established (and if possible, linear) relationship with the change in the clinical status of the skin disease.

Important and desirable characteristics

Objectivity

The lower the dependence of the technique on the 'human element' involved in taking the measurement, the less the opportunity for bias (conscious or unconscious). Clearly the 'nirvana' of robotic measuring devices is some way off, but objectivity can be maintained in the setting of a clinical trial by ensuring that the measurements are taken 'blind'.

Ease and speed of use, robustness, portability and cheapness

If techniques and/or devices for making measurements are difficult to use, cumbersome or expensive, or delicate and keep on breaking down, they will impede the progress of a study and may even destroy it. Such considerations as the number of controls and the visibility of digital displays may dictate the usability of a particular device and hence a particular parameter.

'Useful and interesting' characteristics

This group of characteristics make the life of an investigator easier and more exciting—issues that are not unimportant in ensuring that a trial is successful. They include such factors as the technique providing 'hard copy' of the data rather than a necessity for laboriously writing each datum separately. The provision of data that easily translate into a clinical sign and from there into disease progress also helps the process.

Unaided clinical measurements

It is very difficult to convert subjective clinical observations into measurements that satisfy the requirements stated above. If for reasons of 'convenience', 'economy' or 'conservatism' only clinical observations are to be made, then as many parameters as possible should be evaluated to obtain as much information as possible. The traditional 1–3 scale is often employed. The grades are made to be equivalent to the usual descriptions of 'No change' (0), 'Improved' (+1), 'Much improved' (+2), 'Cleared' (+3) and 'Worse' (−1). Half points are often allowed in this system to account for changes midway between two grades. Although this (and similar systems) is probably the most frequently used of all clinical assessment systems, and it is easy to use and understand, it has several serious disadvantages.

The first of these is that it is a 'short scale', i.e. there are only five points between −1 and +3, and even with half points there are only a limited number of grades that can be allotted to a clinical sign, which makes the system somewhat insensitive to small changes. Even worse than this, the interval between any two adjacent grades is inconstant and not necessarily the same as the interval between any two other adjacent grades. In other words, the difference between 2 and 3 (or for that matter, between 2 and 2.5) may not be the same for Dr Peter as for Dr Paul, or the same for Dr Peter on Tuesday as on Friday, or indeed the same as for the difference between 1 and 2. Thus the scale is not only short and insensitive, its non-equal intervals make it poorly reproducible, non-linear and difficult to analyse.

Some of these difficulties can be surmounted by employing a visual analogue scale in which a mark is made on an unmarked 10 cm long line, the left-hand side of which is zero, indicating the absence of a sign, and the right-hand side of which is 10 indicating the worst possible scenario for the particular feature in question. Such a scale can be used by both physician and patient for virtually any clinical sign or symptom. Measuring the distance from zero to the mark made on the line gives a score. This simple expedient increases the sensitivity of clinical assessment enormously and is surprisingly reproducible in practice. We have

used such scoring systems on many occasions and found them especially useful in the assessment of photodamage.[1]

We have designed and built an electronic visual analogue scale meter where, to save time, the scale is electronic and the measurement read directly by an observer.

Attempts have been made to devise clinical scoring systems for particular disorders that are somewhat less arbitrary because they define points on the severity scale and give guidance on how to use the scale. Such systems include that employed by Cunliffe[2] for acne, which is based on clinical photographs, and that of Frederikson for psoriasis—the psoriasis area and severity index (PASI).[3] In the latter the arms, legs, trunk and head and neck are scored separately for 'area of skin involvement', 'erythema', 'scaling' and 'induration'. Each body part is then 'weighted' and the scores combined using a formula to give an index.

The PASI is a brave attempt at objectifying a series of subjective observations, but in my view falls down on two counts. The first is that it gives equal weight to all physical signs when these do not all have equal biological significance. The second may seem trivial, although in practice it is not—different clinicians have different perceptions as to where different body parts begin and end and are not consistent on the scores they give for the physical signs.[4]

Many of the problems highlighted above can be obviated by adequate planning and training. Good clear definitions and criteria to which all observers agree to adhere, and some training (at a meeting of investigators in multicentre studies) improve the likelihood of detecting a therapeutic response.

Instrumental techniques

Several devices have become available in recent years that make clinical assessment an objective exercise and are sufficiently 'clinician friendly' to be used in the context of a clinical trial.[5] They can be categorized as devices that quantify either a physical sign or a structural feature and devices that measure a physical property or function. There are in addition instruments that record and quantify phenomena that have been found empirically useful, even though it is not certain how the 'phenomena' concerned arise. Measurement of the electrical properties of skin at the skin surface falls into this category. In this brief review it is only possible to mention examples of the many instruments and techniques available and suitable for use in clinical trials. Numerous other devices have been described in the literature.

Measuring physical signs

There is excellent instrumentation available for the measurement of erythema, the degree of pigmentation and the degree of skin thickening. The state of the art is less advanced when it comes to quantifying scaliness and the area of skin involvement. Furthermore, we have scarcely moved off the starting blocks with regard to assessing quantitatively by instrumental means physical signs and disease severity in acne, rosacea, atopic dermatitis or a host of other skin disorders.

Erythema

Our preferred instrument for measurement of erythema is the reflectance spectrophotometer.[6] This device measures the log of the ratio between the absorption of red and green light emitted by modulated light-emitting diodes. The device seems to satisfy the requirements quoted above with regard to repeatability, reproducibility, sensitivity, accuracy, convenience and portability and is already in use in clinical trials.

Pigmentation

A similarly designed reflectance spectrophotometer to the 'erythemameter' has been constructed for the assessment of the degree of pigmentation.[7] This is suitable for measurement of hyperpigmentation of endocrine origin or postinflammatory hyperpigmentation or any other clinical situation in which there is excess melanin pigmentation.

Skin thickening

Pulsed A-scan ultrasound is ideal for measurement of skin thickness[8,9] and has already been used extensively in a variety of clinical studies including evaluation of disease progress in scleroderma[10] and plaque thickness in psoriasis.[11] We believe that ultrasound assessment of plaque thickness is currently the most sensitive technique for assessing the effectiveness of treatment in psoriasis.

Calipers have also been used and, although these are simple, quick and cheap to use, individual readings are much less reliable than those taken with pulsed A-scan ultrasound.

Skin stiffness

The mechanical properties of skin are altered in several disorders, notably systemic sclerosis, the Ehlers–Danlos syndrome and chronic photodamage. Techniques to assess skin stiffness include the uniaxial extensometer[12] and a device that assesses angular deformation after applying a circular torque (the 'Twistometer').[13] Both have been used to assess the effects of treatment on altered mechanical properties of skin.

Scaliness

Measurements of scaling are possible employing optical techniques that assess the shadowing that scales produce when light strikes the skin at an angle. We have used a macrophotographic application of this principle,[14] but until this has been 'packaged' to make it usable in a clinical situation it remains an interesting possibility.

Skin surface contour change has been assessed by submitting replicas to image analytical procedure in the course of trials of tretinoin for photodamage,[15] but this method does not appear to have been used to assess scaling. Anyway, the use of replicas to study scaling is somewhat suspect as the taking of replicas can be considered 'invasive' as far as scaling is concerned.

Area of skin involvement

No satisfactory technique currently exists to assess area of skin involvement apart from in certain specialized situations, e.g. measurement of areas (or volume) of ulceration. Electronic planimetry from standardized photographs and image analytical methods[16] have been attempted, but we are a long way from a clinician friendly measuring device.

Miscellaneous measuring techniques

There are numerous other devices (some commercially available) that are capable of providing assistance with the quantitative assessment of the progress of a skin disorder when being treated in a clinical trial. Measurement of sebum secretion using a lipometer[17] or sebumeter, measurement of the rate of sweat secretion and measurement of the skin's electrical resistance or capacitance[18] are some examples of those available. The choice of the parameter to be studied is the critical issue—many investigations seem just to ignore signs or skin functions that have the potential for making useful clinical measurements.

Conclusion

One of the most important aspects of a clinical trial is the method by which one decides that the trial treatment is more or less successful than 'no treatment' or a competitive treatment. The major theme of this contribution has been that assessment in clinical trials should be quantitative. Many of the techniques and devices for making such measurements already exist and often the only thing lacking is the clinician's willingness to use them.

References

1 Lever L, Kumar P, Marks R, Topical retinoic acid in the treatment of solar elastotic degeneration, *Br J Dermatol* (1990) **122**: 92–8.

2 Cunliffe WJ, Clinical assessment of acne vulgaris, In: *Acne*, London: Martin Dunitz, 1989, Chap. 6, pp. 115–22.

3 Fredriksson T, Pettersson U, Severe psoriasis: oral therapy with a new retinoid, *Dermatologica* (1978) **157**: 238–40.

4 Marks R, Barton S, Shuttleworth D, Finlay A, Assessment of disease progress in psoriasis, *Arch Dermatol* (1989) **125**: 235–40.

5 Marks R, Mechanical properties of the skin. In: Goldsmith LA (ed). *Biochemistry and physiology of the skin*, Oxford: Oxford University Press, 1983, Chap. 57, pp. 1237–54.

6 Pearse AD, Edwards C, Hill S, Marks R, A portable erythema meter and its application to use in human skin, *Int J Soc Cosmet Sci* (1990) **12**: 63–70.

7 Edwards C, Heggie R, A small solid state meter for measuring melanin pigmentation. In: Marks R, Plewig G (eds). *The environmental threat to the skin*, London: Martin Dunitz, 1992, pp. 149–54.

8 Alexander H, Miller DC, Determining skin thickness with pulsed ultrasound, *J Invest Dermatol* (1979) **72**: 17–19.

9 Tan CY, Statham B, Marks R, Payne PA, Skin thickness measurement by pulsed ultrasound: its reproducibility, validation and variability, *Br J Dermatol* (1982) **106**: 657–67.

10 Serup J, Localized scleroderma (morphoea): thickness of sclerotic plaques as measured by 15 MHz pulsed ultrasound, *Acta Derm Venereol (Stockh)* (1984) **64**: 214–19.

11 Khalfan HG, A comparison between clinical, non-invasive instrumental and invasive techniques in assessment of psoriasis, Ph.D. Thesis, University of Wales College of Medicine, Cardiff, 1992.

12 Gunner CW, Williams EW, Greaves M et al, Effects of treatment with prednisolone and PUVA on the mechanical properties of human skin in

vivo. In: Marks R, Payne PA (eds). *Bioengineering and the skin*, Lancaster: MTP Press, 1981, Chap. 5, pp. 31–43.

13 **Kalis B, de Rigal J, Leonard F et al,** *In vivo* study of scleroderma by non-invasive techniques, *Br J Dermatol* (1990) **122**: 785–91.

14 **Marshall RJ, Marks R,** Assessment of skin surface by scanning densitometry of macrophotographs, *Clin Exp Dermatol* (1983) **8**: 121–7.

15 **Grove GL, Grove MJ, Leyden JJ,** Optical profilometry: an objective method for quantification of facial wrinkles, *J Am Acad Dermatol* (1989) **21**: 631–7.

16 **Ramsay B, Lawrence CM,** Measurement of involved surface area in patients with psoriasis, *Br J Dermatol* (1991) **124**: 565–70.

17 **Saint-Leger D, Berrebi C, Duboz C, Agache P,** The lipometre: An easy tool for rapid quantification of skin surface lipids in man, *Arch Dermatol Res* (1979) **265**: 79–89.

18 **Tagami H, Ohi M, Iwatsuki K et al,** Evaluation of the skin surface hydration *in vivo* by electrical measurement, *J Invest Dermatol* (1980) **75**: 500–4.

14

Orphan drugs—the physician's dilemma

Andrew Herxheimer

Introduction

An *orphan drug* is basically a drug that is not commercially viable because the cost of developing it cannot be recovered from sales. Such a drug has no commercial sponsor or adoptive parent, who would apply for a product licence under the Medicines Act. It is therefore liable to remain unlicensed, and outside the normal channels of supply. This creates obvious difficulties for doctors and patients. Before discussing them I should explain three related terms: orphan disease, orphan indication, and orphan dosage. An *orphan disease* is one that is too rare to make it commercially rewarding to develop a treatment for it. A drug which is licensed and available for one or more main indications may have other uses in patients with an orphan disease; this use is then an *orphan indication*. Finally, *orphan dosage* is a new term which refers to the use of a

licensed drug for a licensed indication, but in a dosage differing substantially from that specified in the licence. In the USA, an Orphan Drugs Act was passed in 1983 to facilitate the development and provision of drugs for orphan diseases, and since then the terms 'orphan drug' and 'orphan disease' have been used there in technical legal senses[1] which differ in some ways from those used in this chapter.

In treating a rare disease, using an orphan drug, or using an established drug for an orphan indication, the physician has problems, some of which resemble those faced with any new still unmarketed drug. The central difficulty is a lack of coherent and reliable information: neither a manufacturer nor a regulatory agency has assembled and reviewed the relevant data, and in the case of an orphan treatment, no manufacturer has organized a clinical testing programme. The physician thus carries the responsibility for the treatment alone, although he or she can ask advice from the Medicines Control Agency and from colleagues. The pharmaceutical quality of orphan drugs must also be considered if no accepted standards have been developed.

Orphan drugs

The best known dermatological orphan drug in Britain is *methoxsalen*. It has long been used in ultraviolet radiation (PUVA) treatment for severe psoriasis and mycosis fungoides; the use of PUVA in psoriasis has been studied in many randomized controlled trials and is practised in most skin departments. The fact that methoxsalen is licensed in other countries of the European Community, for example Belgium, Denmark, Germany, Ireland, the Netherlands and Spain, and in Australia, Canada, Switzerland and the USA, suggests a lack of interest amounting to inertia and complacency at the Medicines Control Agency. The Agency is in this instance clearly not doing its job of protecting patients. Methoxsalen *is* mentioned in the *British National Formulary*, but with the caution that it can only be prescribed for named patients, and the *Formulary* does not include a monograph.

A typical example of a relatively new orphan drug is *diphencyprone*, a strong contact allergen which appears to be useful in the treatment of alopecia areata and, possibly, resistant warts. It shows most of the features that characterize an orphan drug: it is not patented and not formulated as a medicine; it has been tried in a relatively small number of heterogeneous patients; it can cause serious adverse effects;[2] and its use requires special experience and circumspection.

After its disastrous short career as a hypnotic, *thalidomide* has in the last few years re-emerged as an orphan drug. Its immunosuppressive activity has been found useful in attenuating acute severe type 2 lepra reactions (erythema nodosum leprosum) and in Behçet's disease. Scattered anecdotal reports of its value in various other rare conditions[3] have given it a somewhat nebulous image of a possible last-resort orphan for these.

Orphan indications

A good example of a drug with many orphan indications is *isotretinoin*, which is licensed only for the treatment of cystic and conglobate acne, and severe acne unresponsive to conventional antimicrobial therapy. It is however also used for less severe cases, for Gram-negative folliculitis, for rosacea that is resistant to long-term tetracycline, and for various rare disorders of keratinization where nothing else seems to help.[4] Very recalcitrant warts and even severe corns have on occasion been treated with the drug.

Cyclosporin is another drug with many orphan indications, most notably psoriasis (the drug is now licensed for use in psoriasis) and atopic eczema. Its use in these conditions is discussed in Chapter 6.

Orphan dosage

My first example also concerns acne. The standard dose of *minocycline* recommended for this purpose by the manufacturer, and specified in the data sheet, is 50 mg twice daily for a minimum of 6 weeks. But some acne patients require 150 or 200 mg a day for 6 months to control their acne

(W. J. Cunliffe, personal communication). It seems that neither the licensing authority nor the manufacturer have taken any notice, let alone done anything in the light of this experience.

A second example of orphan dosage is the antihistamine *terfenadine*, which the manufacturer recommends in a dose of no more than 120 mg a day. It is known that some patients whose symptoms do not respond at this dosage are helped by higher doses. Doses of 180–540 mg daily have been used for urticaria, and to reduce itching in atopic eczema,[5] but such forays into the unknown seem unjustified when well known alternative treatments can be used, especially since high doses can cause ventricular arrhythmias.

The prescriber's dilemma

Now we can consider the doctor's difficulties in using orphan treatment. The prescriber is faced with a patient who cannot be treated adequately by conventional means, and only the use of an orphan treatment appears to offer hope. The doctor has then to rely on published experience with the drug and the condition being treated, and on his or her own previous experience and general knowledge. Published experience, insofar as it exists, is likely to be scattered, hard to assemble, full of holes and often consists of uncontrolled anecdotal observations which cannot be taken at face value. The

Medicines Control Agency cannot or will not help; the manufacturer, if there is one, is reluctant because the law[6] forbids the promotion of any use or dosage outside the terms of the product licence, and the boundary between information and promotion of sales is regarded as a grey area potentially subject to legal dispute. The obvious, and the only practicable solution that I see is collective professional self-help.

Dermatologists can help themselves

I would like to suggest that the specialist association, in this case the British Association of Dermatologists, should take the lead in seeing to the orderly development and use of orphan treatments by dermatologists. This would probably best be done by or under the guidance of a 'Committee for Fostering Orphan Treatments'— COMFORT would be a good optimistic acronym. I would see the committee as eventually having several distinct but related tasks.

1. Early identification of orphan treatments.[7]
2. Design, promotion and performance of controlled trials of the most important of these orphan treatments.[7]
3 Development of one or more standard protocols for the use of each orphan treatment,[7] with the

recommendation that any dermatologist wishing to use the treatment should adhere to it meticulously, and that any proposed modification should be discussed with the appropriate member(s) of the Orphan Treatment Committee before being tried in practice.

4 For each orphan treatment, setting up and maintaining a register of cases treated, with specified clinical details, follow-up and outcomes, including possible adverse effects.

5 Preparation of standard information for patients who are to be offered a particular orphan treatment.

Of course, work of this kind cannot be expected from busy consultants in their spare time, and funding would soon be required for at least one skilled person to coordinate it and its sub-groups. But it should be possible to obtain the relatively modest funds needed through the NHS Research and Development Programme,[8] and perhaps from self-help societies of patients with skin diseases, and research charities related to dermatology.

Such an initiative would have some important advantages.

1. Every patient receiving an orphan treatment would contribute new and valuable knowledge to dermatology, both about benefits and disadvantages.

2. Every dermatologist using an orphan treatment would in so doing make a useful scientific contribution to his/her specialty, and not simply venture forth on unlogged solo patrols into no man's land. I would indeed argue that any prescriber using a new or unexplored treatment is thereby accepting a moral obligation to monitor and record the results.

3. Knowledge about orphan treatments would accrue more quickly and in a more systematic manner; this would make it possible to evaluate them sooner and more reliably than now.

4. It could give dermatologists substantial legal protection against claims of negligence relating to orphan treatments if they could show that they had used the treatment in accordance with standards defined by their peers.

5. It would enhance the scientific standing of the British Association of Dermatologists in Britain and internationally. If the Association were the first specialist association to accept the challenge of dealing constructively with the problem of orphan treatments, it would be a feather in its toupee.

References

1 Lyle WH, Orphan drugs—or orphan diseases? In: Burley D, Haward C, Mullinger B (eds). *The focus for pharmaceutical knowledge*, Macmillan: Basingstoke, 1988, pp. 230–8.

2 de Groot AC, Nater JP, Dermatological drugs, topical agents and cosmetics. In: Dukes MNG, Beeley L

(eds). *Side effects of drugs annual 14*, Elsevier: Amsterdam, 1990, pp. 132–4.

3 Martindale, *The extra pharmacopoeia*, London: Pharmaceutical Press, 29th edn, 1989, pp. 1621–2.

4 Dollery CT (ed), *Therapeutic drugs*, Vol. 1, Edinburgh: Churchill Livingstone, 1991, p. I113.

5 Doherty V, Sylvester DGH, Kennedy CTC et al, Treatment of itching in atopic eczema with antihistamines with a low sedative profile, *Br Med J* (1989) **298**: 96.

6 (UK) Medicines Act 1968, Sections 92ff, London: HMSO.

7 Advisory Group on Health Technology Assessment for the Director of Research and Development, Department of Health, *Assessing the effects of health technologies: principles, practice, proposals*, London: Department of Health, 1992.

8 Department of Health, *Research for health. A research and development strategy for the NHS*, London: HMSO, 1991.

15

Medical ethics—the patient's viewpoint

Carolyn Faulder

I first began investigating clinical trials in 1980 when I was invited to join a working party then preparing the protocol for a new breast cancer randomized clinical trial. Funded by the Cancer Research Campaign, the aim was to measure survival outcomes by comparing mastectomy with lumpectomy in early stage breast cancer. The trial was considered necessary because an earlier, similar trial at Guy's Hospital in London, had been flawed in respect of the adjuvant radiotherapy regime.[1]

The purpose of inviting me onto the working party was to obtain a lay opinion concerning informed consent. The working party was facing a serious dilemma. Should patients always be told they were participating in a trial? More particularly, should they be told about this trial, taking into account all its attendant, and very sensitive, emotional and psychological implications? If so, what should they be told? When, how and by whom was the information to be given?[2]

My qualifications for this task I could only ascribe to having written a chapter about informed consent in my first book on breast cancer.[3] Timid and deferential as I now consider that piece of writing to be, it did signify a personal watershed. I learned that it was one thing to debate the principle of informed consent in learned journals, and quite another to put it into practice.

My further research revealed certain facts about randomized controlled trials which in some respects are unchanged today. They can be summarized under three headings.

1. Randomized control trials were ubiquitous but there was no central coordinating body to register, monitor and log their progress and results.
2. Randomized control trials raised very particular problems, both ethical and practical, regarding informed consent.
3. Few people, apart from the trialists themselves, knew very much about randomized control trials. Furthermore, this state of ignorance (it sometimes looked more like blithe indifference) included many doctors and other health professionals.

What concerned me most at that time, and shocked me when I realized its full importance, was to discover where patients stood in the midst of all this scientific activity. For, if some doctors could be described as woefully ignorant about current medical research, some of those involved in trials appeared to be deliberately imposing ignorance on their patients. They, undoubtedly, would have described their actions more euphemistically, as 'shielding their patients from the unpleasant truth', believing that it was in the patients' best interests not to be overly informed.

The more I investigated, the more apparent it became that there were many patients in general practitioners' surgeries, out-patient clinics and on hospital wards who were participants in randomized control trials, but without their knowledge; therefore, obviously, without their consent. What about the right to know and the right to make informed decisions and choices, which we take for granted in our normal, everyday, healthy lives? Did something happen when one became a patient that removed these rights and, with them, autonomy?

And what about those excellent guidelines for the proper practice of medical research, embodied in the Declaration of Helsinki as long ago as 1964? Clear, comprehensive and, in my view at least, incontrovertible, they were cogently set forth in that document, drawn up by doctors for doctors, and have since been revised and updated on more than one occasion.

My brief is to present the patient's viewpoint. Ten years ago that would have been very difficult. Patients did not have a viewpoint about medical ethics in clinical trials, for the simple reason that they knew next to nothing about them. As a lay person, writing and speaking about informed consent, and the duty to empower patients to use their right to give it, I was sometimes accused of representing only myself plus a tiny minority. This was once memorably characterized by the speaker preceding me at a conference, as 'the archetypal trendy middle class *Guardian* woman reader living in the muesli belt of North London'.

Five years ago, it was already easier to talk about the patient's viewpoint. I knew it was a reality, so I no longer felt like some kind of impostor speaking on behalf of people for whom I had no existential proof. In the early days any evidence I could produce was necessarily anecdotal. However, the feedback from my own work and, more importantly, the respectable body of evidence beginning to emerge from respected academic research, both medical and sociological, made it clear that the principle of 'informed consent' was not a fanciful abstraction, dreamed up to keep philosophers occupied and lawyers in business. Nor was 'patient autonomy' an idle conceit. Patients themselves were beginning to demand more information and were becoming more assertive about their right to make decisions and to be offered choices where possible.

Today, the patient's viewpoint is slowly evolving into a firmer, more informed and ever more confident position. It can no longer be disregarded or brushed aside as being of no consequence. We even have a

'Patients' Charter', produced by the Government no less—not a very impressive document—and there are others. But charters and codes are no more than guidelines, worth less than the paper they are written on, if there is not the will to breathe life into them, and the commitment to follow them through.

Two points must be borne in mind by anyone purporting to represent the patient's view. The first is that patients are all unique individuals, each one coming from a different place and background; each one having a unique life experience and special personal relationships; each one having expectations, values, beliefs and denials, making each one a person like no other person, whether they be whole or damaged or suffering or defeated or fighting. Therefore, any claim to talk about a collective 'patients' viewpoint', must be tempered by acknowledging that important individual differences will always remain.

The second is that any 'viewpoint', whoever's it may be, which is set in a medical ethical context is flexible, and has the possibility of change written into it. Medical ethics is not an absolute and immutable value system, nor does it have rules or laws that can be written in tablets of stone. What we may, today, think to be the only right and proper course of action in a given set of circumstances may, tomorrow, be nullified by unforeseen factors: for example, a startling development in medical technology—say some extraor-

dinary new life-saving or life-changing technique—may force society to develop, modify or alter its moral stance in some important respect. These situations are already occurring.

Certain values, however, we must hope will not change. Among these are the doctors' duty of care towards their patients which, as I understand it, means always to act in the patient's best interests, even if that best can sometimes amount to no more than doing them as little harm as possible. No less important in the context of medical ethics, is the respect for a patient's autonomy which should only be overruled in exceptional and quite dire circumstances.

Just as the collective 'patients' viewpoint' has changed over the past decade, so, in a different time-scale, has the individual's viewpoint evolved within the patient–doctor relationship. Although the patient's viewpoint has its initial springboard in the patient's own psyche, its ultimate crystallization depends very crucially on how that relationship—with the doctor, primarily, but with other health carers too— has developed: whether it has been rooted in a fruitful, expanding dialogue, or whether it has become stunted or distorted for any number of reasons, some not hard to imagine.

An evolutionary process implies a sequence of transformations, each following and merging into one another, apparently imperceptibly. Nonetheless, it is usually possible to observe major cut-off and start-up points. Where the patient is concerned, three distinct stages can be observed. They are 'expectation', 'understanding' and 'participation'.

The patient's expectation starts at the moment when the patient, aware of a problem, presents himself or herself to the doctor. He or she is there, in the surgery or clinic, because it is his or her belief that the doctor is the expert: the person equipped by training and experience to diagnose and treat the problem. The patient hopes for cure, or at the least, alleviation of the problem.

In this first expectant (and naive) stage, the only ethical dimension that most patients are aware of is that the doctor must care for them to the best of his or her ability. The patient trusts the doctor so to do and perceives ethical responsibility, probably defined as good and/or kind behaviour, to be entirely on the side of the doctor.

Soon, though, the patient begins to 'wise up' as the doctor starts to explain the diagnosis and proposed treatment, or, conversely, the impossibility of making a hard and fast diagnosis, at least immediately. The benefits and disadvantages of various treatments are discussed, and symptoms, side-effects, outcomes, all begin to figure in further talks.

The patient enters the second stage—understanding; this may arise slowly and reluctantly, or in leaps and bounds. Much depends on the nature of the information being imparted, and much too on the doctor's communication skills. A lot also depends on the patient's readiness to know, and willingness to be involved. This understanding can, of course, be encouraged or retarded, depending on the quality of the dialogue between patient and doctor.

The medical dimension is only part of it. Understanding is on many levels and comes in many ways. It may be a straightforward acquisition of factual information which the patient then sets about adapting to; it may be a subtle intuitive perception, for example, of the implications of the illness on the patient's personal life; or it may come through a ravaging emotional onslaught, anger, for instance, or grief or fear. By whatever route understanding enters the patient's mind, it will infiltrate many areas of the patient's life about which the doctor knows nothing or, at best, can only hazard a guess. Inevitably, as the patient's understanding of the situation grows, it will have a potent effect on the patient's viewpoint.

Most patients gradually become aware that there are few simple or certain answers in medicine. Doubt enters the picture; so too, does the spectre of failure. Choice may become a real possibility. But the existence of choice can be confusing and mean that difficult decisions may have to be made. The patient's growing understanding of the situation can obviously stir up serious concerns. 'I didn't expect to be told that they didn't know the best treatment for me. It was left to me to decide what I wanted', can be a cry of despair, not a shout for independence.

Other patients will feel relieved, even pleased, as they realize that being invited to discuss choices allows them to recover some control of their lives. They welcome the chance to share the decision-making with their doctor, and they appreciate that the burden of ethical responsibility should not have to lie with the doctor alone.

Some patients will still want to say 'I leave it all to you, you know best', but I suspect this is a shrinking group. And it may become more difficult in the future for them to do so, as increasing numbers of doctors feel uneasy about bearing the burden alone, and not simply for ethical reasons. The threat of a malpractice suit is a growing cloud on the horizon.

The third-stage patient has come a long way. No longer so oppressed by a sense of inferiority and helplessness—mainly due to knowing so little—he or she can now feel, with some justification, that he or she is an equal partner, genuinely participating in the joint enterprise of healing. As such the patient fully shares with the doctor a sense of personal responsibility for the choices made and decisions taken. Trust, that vital bond between patient and doctor, on which both rightly lay so much store, is consolidated.

Patient and doctor may not always be in agreement, but in a mature relationship each should have respect and consideration for the other's point of view, including any ethical issues where they may appear to be at variance. For instance, a patient may want a treatment which the doctor may feel unhappy about for good medical, and/or ethical, reasons. Conversely, a patient may refuse a treatment for reasons which the doctor finds unreasonable. Each side must be willing to hear the other out. Listening is an essential part of their dialogue.

Integral to the formation of a 'patient's viewpoint' along the lines I have described, is the tacit assumption that no decisions will be taken without fully involving and informing the patient. Consent will only be sought when both patient and doctor feel that adequate information has been imparted and the patient allowed enough time to discuss and consider the implications.

To do so, acknowledges the respect that the doctor, and everyone else, has for the patient's autonomy. Secondly, it furthers the important aim, now generally recognized as one to strive for, to help as many patients as possible to become active, intelligent participants in their treatment. Leaving ethics on one side, this also happens to make sound clinical sense. Research shows that not only are informed patients more cooperative, they also do better and make a speedier recovery, than the passive, ignorant patient who is often unaware, for instance, of the importance of compliance.

I would like to suggest that we should regard 'informed consent' as having two aspects: it is both a principle and a process. In the context of a clinical trial it remains no less essential to view informed consent as a principle that cannot be jettisoned, however awkward it may be sometimes to put into practice. In a randomized control trial the eligible patient has a right to be fully informed about the trial *before* randomization into groups takes place, and to decide at that preliminary stage whether he or she wishes to participate. It is not, therefore, ethically acceptable first to enter the patients and then to tell them about the trial, because this is not giving them complete information. They may well not realize, for instance, that they could have been randomized to another group, and this matters. The doctor giving the information also must be careful not to sound too persuasive. There is always the danger, human nature being what it is, that an element of coercion creeps into the situation. The patient could be afraid of 'letting the doctor down' or 'making the doctor angry' by refusing consent, or even that he or she will not be looked after so well.

The doctor is obliged to put his or her clinical responsibility for the individual patient before personal research interests or the interests of colleagues or other parties. This means that if a patient has difficulty understanding the nature and purpose of the trial, it may not be possible to ask for that patient's consent. Or, if it seems a patient might find the terms of partici-

pation unacceptable, it is not ethical to brush over certain aspects of the trial, e.g. the need to randomize.

On the patient's side, competence (to understand what is being proposed) and voluntariness (the freedom to say yes or no without fear of retribution) are obviously essential for a valid informed consent.

The 'viewpoints' of both parties are dependent on many factors beyond the relatively restricted medical arena and they are always susceptible to new influences. If the duality of informed consent is recognized as a constant element in the continuing dialogue between patient and doctor, the resulting improved understanding on both sides can only be of mutual benefit.

References

1 Hayward JL, The Guy's trial of treatments of early breast cancer, *World J Surg* (1977) **11**: 314–18.

2 Cancer Research Campaign Working Party in Breast Conservation, Informed consent: ethical, legal and medical implications for patients and doctors who participate in randomised clinical trials, *Br Med J* (1983) **286**: 1117–21.

3 Faulder C, *Breast cancer—a guide to its early detection and treatment*, London: Pan, 1979. (Superseded by *The women's cancer book*, London: Virago, 1989.)

16

Surgical treatments

The cutting edge

Clifford Lawrence

Introduction

Dermatological surgery therapy should be sufficient to effect cure without the creation of unnecessary scarring or disfigurement. This guiding principle should be applied to the surgical management of both benign and malignant skin lesions by all dermatologists. This chapter highlights techniques that achieve this objective and briefly describes the consequences of aspirin and non-steroidal anti-inflammatory drug (NSAID) therapy in dermatological surgery patients.

The treatment of skin tumours

Mohs surgery for non-melanoma skin cancer results in complete excision of the tumour with minimal removal of normal surrounding tissue, creating a smaller defect, and hence a less complex repair and potentially better cosmetic result than conventional surgery. This benefit of Mohs surgery is well demonstrated in a study of 22 patients with basal cell carcinomas

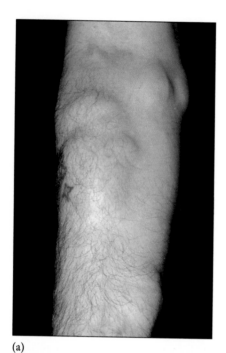

(a)

Figure 16.1

Removal of multiple lipomas through 4 mm punch biopsy wounds. (a) Prior to surgery. (b) Removal of the lipoma through the 4 mm punch biopsy site after the fat had been broken up by blunt dissection.

(b)

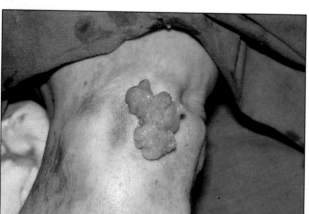

around the eye.[1] An oculoplastic surgeon examined and predicted the size and nature of the repair required to close the anticipated defect that would be left if the tumours were excised using accepted excision margins; the tumours, however, were excised using Mohs horizontal

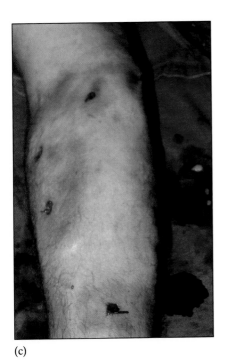

(c)

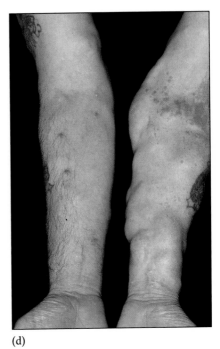

(d)

(c) Immediate post-operative site showing the punch biopsy wounds and extensive bruising caused by strenuous squeezing and manipulation of the lipoma. (d) Two months after removal of multiple lipomas through seven punch biopsy wounds the small scars and relatively normal forearm contour can be seen and compared to the still-affected opposite arm.

sections. As a result of the preservation of normal tissue, the closure of the defect was significantly less extensive than anticipated in over 40% of cases. More importantly, if these tumours had been excised using the margins predicted by the oculoplastic surgeons, it was estimated from the shape of the final defect that over 60% of the tumours would have been incompletely excised. While studies such as these and large published series from enthusiasts suggest that the results of Mohs surgery are superior to all others, sceptics will never be convinced until prospective randomized studies of the results and resources required for plastic surgery compared with Mohs surgery excision of large and recurrent non-melanoma skin cancer become available. Without such studies it seems unlikely that the technique will become generally accepted in the UK by non-dermatologists.

The treatment of benign lesions

Lipomas

Soft mobile lipomas can be expressed through tiny excisions without the need to make a large incision the complete length of the lipoma (Fig. 16.1). A 4 mm punch biopsy hole is made through the skin over the centre of the lump. The lipoma can be broken up by blunt dissection, using artery forceps, and the fragments squeezed out through the 4 mm hole. Alternatively the lipoma can be broken up and sucked out using the liposuction technique.

Epidermoid cysts

Large epidermoid cysts can be managed in a similar way. A 3–4 mm punch biopsy hole is made through the skin over the cyst, to include the cyst punctum if present, and the contents expressed. The cyst size is thus greatly decreased and in non-inflamed cysts the collapsed cyst wall may be removed through the 4 mm excision at this stage. Because the cyst wall tears easily in inflamed or fibrotic cysts complete removal can be delayed to allow the inflammation to subside before attempting complete cyst wall removal; the punch biopsy site does not require sutures. After 4–6 weeks a 1 cm or less incision is made through the punch biopsy site, the cyst wall identified and removed by blunt dissection.

Steatocystoma multiplex

Similar techniques have recently been described for the management of steatocystoma multiplex.[2] Small stab incisions are made over the cysts to be removed. The cyst wall can be grasped through the wound with forceps and pulled through the skin. Each of these techniques avoids the need for long incisions and the subsequent larger scars and stitch marks; this is particularly important in benign conditions in which multiple lesions occur throughout life.

Chondrodermatitis nodularis

On the helix and anti-helix, only cartilage needs to be removed to cure chondrodermatitis nodularis. On the helix an incision is made along the helical rim and the underlying cartilage exposed. A thin slice of cartilage is then removed with the lesion at the centre and the skin edges sutured. On the anti-helix a flap of skin has to be lifted in order to expose sufficient cartilage to allow the damaged areas of cartilage to be excised. The exposed cartilage is excised taking great care to leave no rough cartilage edges and the skin sutured back into place. In a series of 46 cases, 90% of lesions on

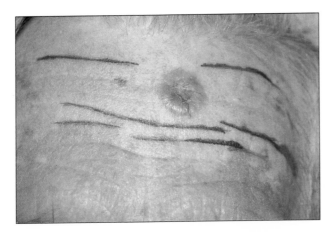

Figure 16.2

Basal cell carcinoma on the forehead showing preoperative marking of the large skin crease lines.

the helix and 70% of those on the anti-helix healed and remained healed for between 4.5–34 months (mean 16 months) when treated in this way.[3] The technique clarifies the principle of therapy and has the advantage that, as so little tissue is removed, the ear shape is preserved; if recurrences occur further similar procedures can be performed without distorting the shape of the ear.

Elliptical excision vs dog ear repair

In small excisions the direction and length of the final scar are anticipated by the surgeon who designs an elliptical shaped excision the direction of which is based on the operator's expertise and local anatomy. The excision length is determined by the time honoured advice that the wound

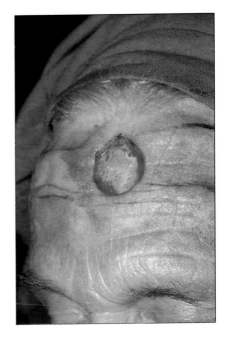

Figure 16.3

Defect after excision of the tumour with an appropriate margin of normal skin.

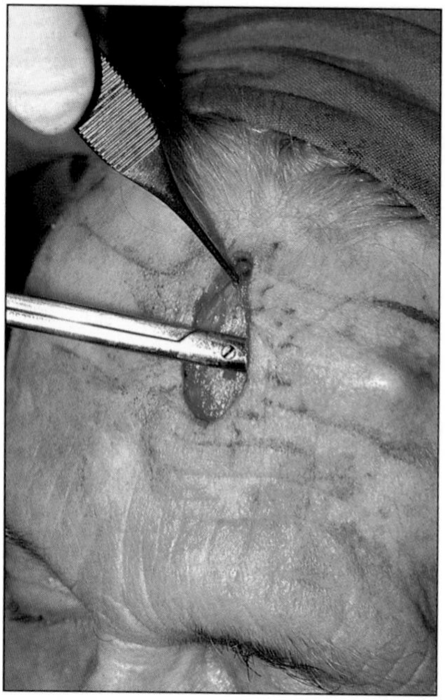

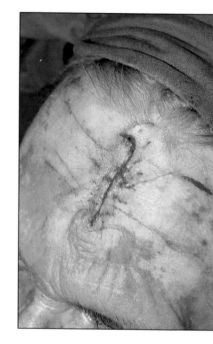

Figure 16.4

Undermining the defect below the frontalis muscle and above the periosteum.

Figure 16.5

Closure was possible using the tissue mobility gained by undermining. The scar could be placed parallel to the frown lines. The skin edges have been apposed using an absorbable Vicryl suture and a dog-ear created by closure of the oval defect can be seen at the lower pole. The dog-ear repair at the upper pole has been started.

length should be approximately three times as long as the width. This technique has the merit of simplicity and speed and on wrinkled skin the optimum scar direction is usually readily identified, although the final scar may be unnecessarily long. By contrast on non-wrinkled skin and the limbs and trunk the ellipse direction anticipated by the surgeon is often not optimal and does not run completely parallel to the relaxed skin tension lines (Fig. 16.2). In general, for all except the smallest excisions, elliptical excisions should be avoided. Instead the lesion should be excised with an

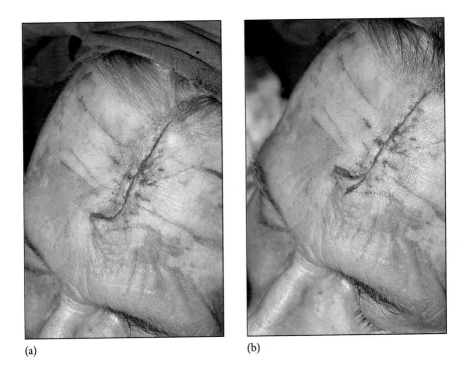

(a)   (b)

Figure 16.6

Starting the dog-ear repair at the lower pole (a), completion of the repair (b), and
the triangular shape of the piece of skin removed (c) *(contd p. 116)*.

appropriate margin of uninvolved skin;
this will leave an oval or circular defect
which should then be closed at the
centre, possibly creating dog-ears at
the corners of the wound which can be
removed if necessary. The resulting
scar is smaller than would be created
by elliptical excision; at some sites the
wound edges can be sutured without
dog-ear formation due to natural skin
tension, thus further minimizing the
length of the scar. Furthermore, the
possibility of a poorly orientated scar is
minimized since the operator is not
committed to placing the final closure
in any particular direction until all
possible wound closure directions have
been assessed. In most cases the direction of the final scar will be determined by the longitudinal axis of the
oval shape created by the interaction of
the shape excised and the shape
produced by the effects of natural skin
tension lines. This allows natural skin

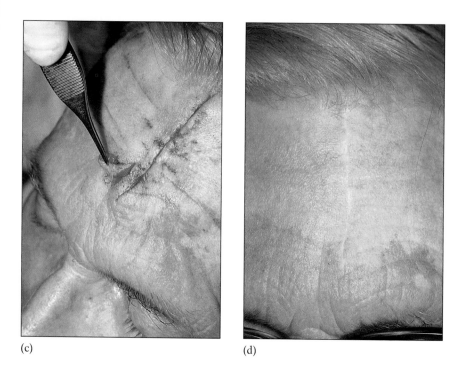

(c)   (d)

Figure 16.6 *continued*

Incision lines are made or scored using the scalpel, but the cutting is done with
sharp scissors. The final wound edges were closed with a running subcuticular suture
which was removed at 8 days. (d) Cosmetic result 1 year later.

tension to create an oval from a circular shaped excision, the long axis of
which lies parallel to the natural skin
tension lines (Figs 16.3 to 16.6).
Comparison of the final excision
length after defect closure and dog-ear
repair compared with the theoretical
length of an elliptical excision of the
same defect, based on the 3:1 ratio,
shows that after dog-ear closure the
scar length was over 20% shorter than

the predicted elliptical closure length
(Hudson-Peacock and Lawrence,
unpublished data).

Second intention healing

Fred Mohs gave his name to the idea
of complete tumour removal with
minimal normal tissue excision and
also demonstrated and championed the

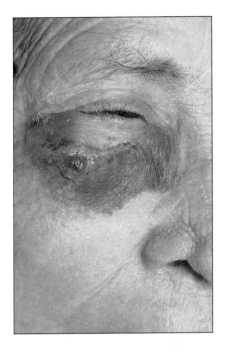

Figure 16.7

Extensive preoperative subcutaneous bleeding in a patient after local anaesthetic injection. This patient was taking aspirin prior to operation, although this did not become apparent until after local anaesthetic injection when extensive subcutaneous bleeding occurred. The operation was cancelled and the aspirin withdrawn for 7 days before attempting tumour excision.

excellent cosmetic results achieved by second intention healing at selected sites after skin tumour excision.[4] Second intention healing should also be considered in the management of benign conditions. Elliptical excisions for moles on the back frequently leave a large stretched scar with parallel stitch marks. If such moles are excised using an oval or circular excision and the defect allowed to heal by second intention, the subsequent scar is smaller than the original wound because approximately 45% of wound healing occurs by scar shrinkage,[5] there are no stitch marks, and because the scar is oval or round it blends more readily with other associated natural defects or scars on the back.[6]

On the ear after excision of basal cell, but not squamous cell, carcinomas which invade cartilage, it is possible to remove the tumour exposing the underlying perichondrium. The defect can then be allowed to heal by second intention. In order to reduce the risk of cartilage desiccation and subsequent necrosis the rate of healing can be increased by placing multiple 2–3 mm punch biopsies through the cartilage, thus allowing granulation tissue to migrate from the back of the ear through the perforated cartilage and cover the perichondrium more rapidly than would be produced from the skin edge alone.[7]

The effect of aspirin and NSAID therapy on bleeding problems in dermatological surgery

Patients taking aspirin or NSAIDs are normally considered to be more likely to bleed freely at operation due to the fact that these drugs inhibit platelet aggregation. In practice, most derma-

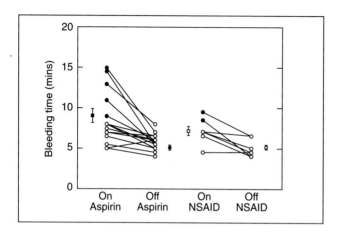

Figure 16.8

Effect of aspirin and NSAID therapy on bleeding time in dermatological surgery patients. A total of 16 patients taking aspirin and 7 taking NSAIDs stopped treatment for a minimum of 5 days prior to surgery. The mean ±SEM (■ and bars) bleeding time on aspirin (mean 9 min) compared with off aspirin (mean 5 min) was highly significant ($p<0.001$, paired Student's t-test), although only five patients (●) had a prolonged bleeding time on aspirin (normal range (shown by stippled area) 2–8 min). The mean ±SEM (□ and bars) bleeding time on NSAIDs (mean 7 min) compared with off NSAIDs (mean 5 min) was highly significant ($p<0.001$, paired Student's t-test), although only two patients (●) had a prolonged bleeding time on therapy.

tologists ask such patients to stop aspirin or NSAIDs a week before surgery (Fig. 16.7). In an attempt to determine how common bleeding is in such patients and to try to identify those at risk, we examined the bleeding times of patients on and off such therapy and have operated on patients taking aspirin and NSAIDs in order to observe the frequency of bleeding complications.[8] A total of 31 patients receiving aspirin and 18 taking NSAIDs were investigated. The bleeding time dropped significantly ($p<0.001$, paired Student's t-test) from 9 min on aspirin to a mean of 5 min off aspirin (normal range 2–8 min) in 17 patients in whom aspirin was stopped for at least 5 days before surgery, although on aspirin the bleeding time was prolonged in only six of these subjects (Fig. 16.8). In 14 patients

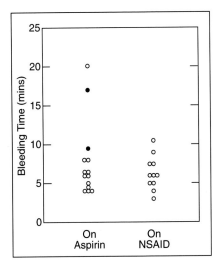

Figure 16.9

Bleeding complications after operating on patients taking aspirin and NSAIDs. Dermatological surgical procedures included tumour excision (16 patients), Mohs excision (5 patients) with delayed repair, punch biopsy (1 patient), excision of cartilage for chondrodermatitis nodularis (2 patients), and curettage of seborrhoeic warts (1 patient). Operations were prolonged or disrupted by excessive bleeding in only two patients (●) taking aspirin, both of whom had prolonged bleeding times. Other patients (○) had normal controllable bleeding.

operations were performed without stopping aspirin therapy (Fig. 16.9). Controllable but increased bleeding occurred in one patient (bleeding time 9.5 min) and in one other patient (bleeding time 17 min) there was uncontrollable bleeding resulting in a greatly prolonged operation, the need

for a pressure dressing and the patient being admitted for observation.

The mean bleeding time dropped significantly ($p<0.001$, paired Student's t-test) from 7 to 5 min when NSAIDs were stopped for a minimum of 5 days in seven patients, although only two patients had a bleeding time outside the normal range (Fig. 16.8). In 11 patients (bleeding time: range 3–10.5 min, mean 6 min) operations were performed whilst the patient was still taking the NSAID. No patient showed increased or uncontrollable bleeding, although two patients had bleeding times greater than 8 min. Thus, in summary, difficulty with haemostasis occurred in less than 15% of patients taking aspirin; preliminary results suggest that these susceptible patients can be identified by their very prolonged bleeding time (Sakuntabhai, Tiling-Grosse and Lawrence, unpublished observations). No conclusion can be drawn about the effect of NSAID therapy as only a small group of patients was studied, although these results suggest that bleeding problems are even less likely in this group.

References

1 **Downes RN, Walker NPJ, Conlin JRO,** Micrographic (Mohs') surgery in the management of periocular basal cell epitheliomas, *Eye* (1990) **4:** 160–8.

2 **Keefe M, Leppard BJ, Royle G,** Successful treatment of steatocystoma multiplex by simple surgery, *Br J Dermatol* (1992) **127:** 41–4.

3 **Lawrence CM,** The treatment of chondrodermatitis nodularis with cartilage removal alone, *Arch Dermatol* (1991) **127:** 530–5.

4 **Mohs FE,** *Chemosurgery. Microscopically controlled surgery for skin cancer,* Springfield, Il: Charles C. Thomas, 1978.

5 **Lawrence CM, Dahl MGC, Comaish JS,** Excision of skin malignancies without wound closure, *Br J Dermatol* (1986) **115:** 563–71.

6 **Barnett R, Strank M,** A method of producing improved scars following excision of small lesions on the back, *Ann Plast Surg* (1985) **3:** 391–4.

7 **James MP,** Multiple cartilage puncture: an aid to second intention healing of defects on the ear, *Br J Dermatol* (1992) **127** (Suppl. 40): 33 (Abstr).

8 **Tiling-Grosse S, Lawrence CM,** Influence of aspirin and NSAID therapy on bleeding time in dermatological surgical patients, *Zentralblatt Haut-und Geschlechtskrankheiten* (1991) **159:** 335 (Abstr).

17

Dermabrasion

Stephen H. Mandy

Introduction

The basic principal of dermabrasion is a rapidly rotating wire brush, or diamond fraise, skillfully applied to the chilled skin. It is recognized as an effective form of therapy for a wide range of indications.[1] It is essential to understand the basic macroscopic anatomy of the skin in order to apply the techniques of dermabrasion which will yield beneficial results. Most important in dermabrasion is the dermis, which is composed basically of two layers, the more superficial papillary layer, and the deeper reticular layer. Injury to the epidermis and papillary dermis heals without scarring, whereas injury which extends into the reticular dermis always results in scar tissue. The goal of all dermabrasive surgery is to reorganize or restructure the collagen of the papillary dermis without resulting in injury to the reticular dermis. The thickness of these dermal layers varies greatly from one area of the skin to another, and while all areas may be dermabraded without scarring it is the face which is ideally

suited to dermabrasion without resultant scar. This is, in part, due to the manner in which dermabrasion wounds heal. Re-epithelialization begins from the wound margins, and from within epidermal appendages which remain following dermabrasion. The pilosebaceous follicle is the primordial germ for this re-epithelialization and the face is richly endowed with sebaceous glands.

The preoperative application of tretinoin (0.05%) for several weeks prior to partial thickness dermabrasive wounds has been shown, both clinically and in the laboratory, to accelerate healing.[2,3] Patients placed on tretinoin prior to dermabrasion will heal in 5–7 days, as contrasted to patients without pretreatment, who heal in 7–10 days (Fig. 17.1). Another

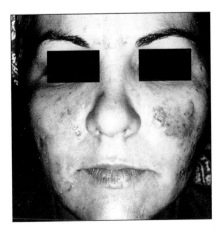

Figure 17.1

Five days after dermabrasion. The patient's right side was pretreated with tretinoin; the left was untreated.

significant factor in promoting healing of dermabrasive wounds is the use of occlusive dressings. Since the work of Maibach and Rovee,[4] it has been well understood that wounds which are treated by occlusive dressings heal up to 40% faster than wounds left to air dry. This is especially true with dermabrasive wounds which when covered with appropriate biosynthetic dressings heal much more rapidly than those left to form crusts.[5] Furthermore, the biosynthetic dressings alleviate postoperative pain almost immediately upon their application following surgery. Biosynthetic dressings act to keep wounds moist, thereby allowing free epithelial migration across the surface. They also cause wound fluids (which contain growth factors that stimulate wound healing) to remain in constant contact with the wound's surface. There is also increasing laboratory evidence to suggest that the presence of an occlusive dressing modulates collagen synthesis and results in a cosmetically more satisfying scar.[6]

Patient selection and indications

Among the many indications for dermabrasion, those most common today are the treatment of acne scars, facial wrinkles, premalignant solar keratoses, rhinophyma, traumatic and surgical scars, and tattoos. Acne scars represent the single greatest application of the dermabrasive technique.

Dramatic improvement may be achieved with facial scarring due to acne, but perfection is impossible. Patients must be given very realistic expectations of the results that surgery can achieve. In patients that have very deep ice-pick-type scarring, punch excision followed by suture closure of the scars 4–6 weeks prior to dermabrasion is most likely to yield a good result. Patients who have extensive acne scarring should be warned of the possibility of further scarring as a result of dermabrasion. Patients with dark pigmentation should be warned of the possibility of hypo- or hyperpigmentation postoperatively. Most frequently, this is transitory and pigment returns to normal over the course of several months. Occasionally, if the scarring is deep, and consequently dermabrasion is deep, pigmentation may be altered permanently. This is especially likely in patients of oriental extraction.

Today, we frequently encounter patients for dermabrasion who have been treated for their acne with systemic 13-*cis*-retinoic acid. This potent antiacne agent causes sebaceous gland atrophy, and from the early days of its use concern was expressed that it might delay wound healing in dermabrasion patients. Initial reports in the literature indicated that dermabrasion patients were unaffected by previous treatment with oral isotretinoin.[7] However, later reports suggested that patients who had been dermabraded following oral isotretinoin therapy exhibited atypical scarring post-

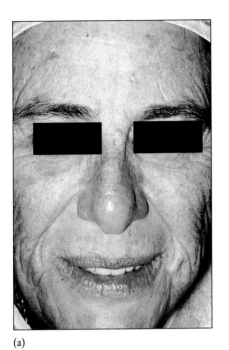

(a)

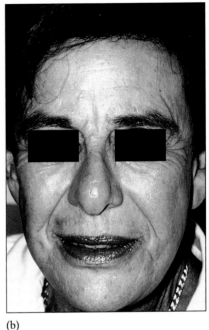

(b)

Figure 17.2

(a) Rhagades and solar keratoses before dermabrasion. (b) Six months after dermabrasion.

dermabrasion.[8] Subsequent to those reports, other authors have reported on numerous patients who have been treated with oral isotretinoin and then dermabraded without sequelae.[9] This unsettling controversy clearly has significant medical and legal implications. A clear-cut cause-and-effect relationship has not, at this time, been established between oral isotretinoin and atypical scarring. Conversely, laboratory studies have failed to substantiate any abnormalities in fibroblast activities or collagen synthesis in the skin of patients treated with oral isotretinoin.[10,11] Until an answer to this question is found, it is probably prudent for physicians to suggest that oral isotretinoin treated patients should wait at least 6 months before undergoing a dermabrasion.

The AIDS virus has been the latest factor to consider when selecting patients for dermabrasion. Of all

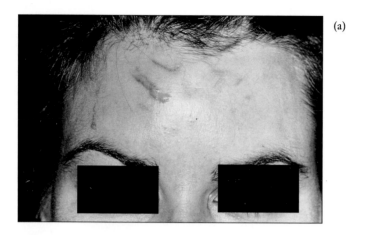

(a)

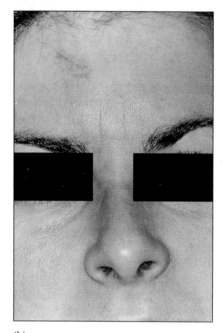

(b)

Figure 17.3

(a) A 6-week-old traumatic scar. (b) The scar 1 month after dermabrasion.

surgeries performed, dermabrasion is most likely to produce an aerosol of blood and tissue products as well as live infective virus particles. A recent study by Wentzell et al[12] indicated that aerosol particles produced during dermabrasion were of sufficient size to allow for access to, and retention by, mucosal and pulmonary surfaces. Furthermore, the study indicated that commonly used personal protection standards such as operatory masks, goggles, and scatter shields, do not prevent the inspiration of these particles. In addition, the settling velocities of such small particles may extend the exposure for many hours after the procedure has been performed, thereby endangering personnel not directly involved in the procedure itself. Another problem which the AIDS virus may cause is the inability to determine if a patient is in a latent period between infection and positive antibody test. It is quite clear that a risk to the physician, his or her

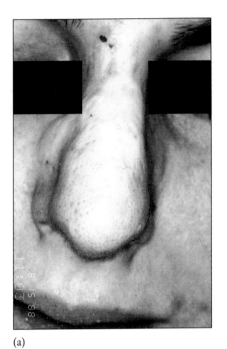

(a)

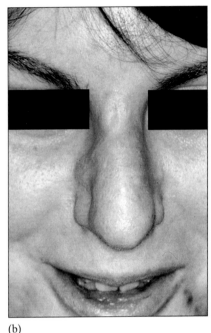

(b)

Figure 17.4

(a) Surgical scar before dermabrasion. (b) The scar after dermabrasion and the use of occlusive dressings.

assistants and other personnel does exist. Dermabrasion certainly should not be performed without a thorough history of high risk behavior, protection of gloves, masks, and goggles, and the awareness that even with such protective devices a certain degree of risk remains.

One of the growing indications for dermabrasion is aging skin, especially that which has been actinically damaged and shows pathology such as premalignant solar keratoses. Dermabrasion has been shown to be effective, if not more so, than topically applied 5-fluorouracil in the management of precancerous skin lesions.[13] In a study of half-face planing of actinically damaged skin, Burke et al[14] showed that precancerous lesions were substantially reduced and their future development retarded over a 5-year period. These factors, combined with the dramatic improvement in rhagades

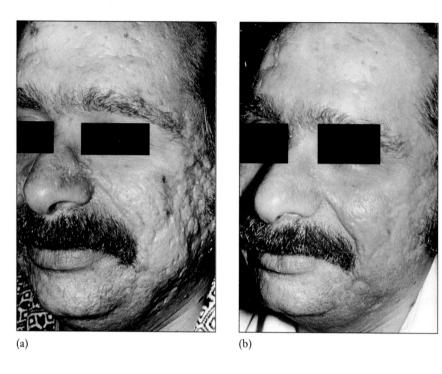

(a)   (b)

Figure 17.5

(a) Acne scars before dermabrasion. (b) The scars after dermabrasion.

seen in dermabrasion patients, make dermabrasion a viable modality in the treatment of aging skin (Fig. 17.2).

Yarborough[15] demonstrated that dermabrasion performed on traumatic or surgical scars approximately 6 weeks after injury often results in the complete disappearance of the scars (Fig. 17.3). In my experience, surgical scars respond so well to dermabrasion that most patients who have had excisional surgery are told that it is likely they may have a dermabrasion 6 weeks postoperatively. Although this is usually not necessary, its anticipation by the patient eases introduction to such treatment when necessary. This is especially true in patients who have very greasy skin or in facial areas such as the nose where improvement following dermabrasion is most dramatic. The improvement in scars following dermabrasion is further enhanced by the postoperative use of biosynthetic dressings which have been demonstrated to significantly affect collagen synthesis, resulting in cosmetic improvement in the surgical scar[6] (Fig. 17.4).

Removal of tattoos can be accomplished with superficial dermabrasion, followed by application of 1% gentian violet and a vaseline gauze dressing daily for 10 days. The gentian violet delays healing, causing the pigment to leach out into the dressing and creating continued inflammation which causes phagocytosis of the pigment. Care to abrade only to the very upper papillary dermis will avoid scarring. Removal of the pigment by abrasion should not be attempted. Professional tattoos are more responsive to such treatment than amateur or traumatic tattoos, but all can be improved. Usually, 50% resolution can be achieved with one procedure, which can be repeated every 2–3 months until the desired result is achieved. Tattoos are a very good training procedure for the novice in dermabrasion.

Benign tumours such as adenoma sebaceum and syringomas may be successfully dermabraded with marked cosmetic improvement, but gradual recurrence is the usual outcome. Dramatic improvement may be achieved with rhinophyma when dermabrasion is combined with electrofulguration (Fig. 17.5).

Instrumentation

A wide variety of abrading instruments have been developed and are commercially available. They vary from hand engines, to cable-driven power sources and battery-operated units. The important consideration in terms of the power source is that it has the torque necessary to continue a sustained and even drive of the abrading surface, either a wire brush or a diamond fraise. The excellent reviews by Yarborough[16] and Alt[17] of the wire brush and diamond fraise dermabrasive techniques require little elaboration. It cannot be overemphasized, however, that no instrument can be substituted for thorough hands-on experience in a preceptorship environment, where the student is able to watch and assist someone experienced in the art of dermabrasion. Most authors agree that the wire-brush technique requires more skill and runs a higher risk of potential injury, as it can cut much deeper and much more quickly than the diamond fraise. In my opinion, with the possible exception of the extra-coarse diamond fraise, superior results are achieved with the wire brush. One of the current controversies surrounding dermabrasion surgery is the use of preabrasive chilling of the skin. Animal and clinical work on various cryaesthesic materials available to chill the skin prior to sanding have shown that use of materials which freeze the skin below $-30°C$, and more especially below $-60°C$, involves the risk of causing substantial tissue necrosis and subsequent scarring.[18–20] It is necessary to freeze the skin prior to dermabrasion in order to have a rigid surface which will abrade evenly, and to preserve anatomic markings which might otherwise be distorted when the tissue has thawed. Since thermal injury may result in excessive scarring, caution would suggest that using cryaesthetic agents which do not freeze below −30°C is prudent and as effective as using those which freeze deeper.

Technique

Preoperative staged analgesia has made dermabrasion a feasible technique for an out-patient setting. Diazepam administered approximately 45 min to 1 h preoperatively, in conjunction with 0.4 mg of atropine intramuscularly as an amnestic and antivagal agent, tend to make the patient more comfortable and less anxious. Prior to administering regional block anesthesia with a Xylocaine–bipuvocaine mixture, 1 cm^3 of intravenously administered Fentanyl gives the patient a great sense of euphoria, while relieving the discomfort associated with regional anesthesia. Fentanyl offers the advantages of being rapid in onset and very short in duration, thus allowing most patients to completely recover from its effect within 30–45 min. Once Fentanyl has taken effect, the administration of the regional anesthesia to the supraorbital, infraorbital, and mental foramina usually results in anesthesia to 60–70% of the face. When this is coupled with the use of the refrigerant spray, most patients can be dermabraded without pain. The use of nitrous oxide analgesia to supplement anesthesia if the patient becomes uncomfortable during the procedure allows the procedure to progress without interruption. Once the skin has been rendered solid by the refrigerant spray, the sanding procedure is begun in areas no larger than that which can be abraded in approximately 10 s, or approximately 1 in^2 areas. The dermabrasion instrument, which should be grasped firmly in the hand, should be pulled only in the direction of the handle and perpendicular to the plane of rotation — back and forth, or circular movements may gouge the skin. The wire brush in particular requires almost no pressure, and produces multiple microlacerations which are a sign of the adequacy of the depth of the procedure. Adequate depth is recognized by several landmarks as one progresses through the skin. The removal of skin pigmentation signifies passage through the basal layer of the epidermis. As one advances into the papillary dermis, the small capillary loops of the papillary plexus are identified as the tissue thaws and punctate bleeding results. As the papillary dermis is entered further, faintly visible, small parallel strands of collagen become apparent. It is the fraying of these parallel strands that signifies that dermabrasion is carried to the correct level — going further may result in scarring.

Many authors suggest the use of cotton towels or cotton gloves as absorbent material for blotting instead of using gauzes which may become ensnared in the dermabrading instruments. The entanglement of gauze in the instruments results in a loud flapping which both frightens the patient and may often compromise the function of the instrument itself.

In my experience, it is easiest to begin the dermabrasion centrally beside the nose and work outwards, as the area around the nose is usually the area of greatest disfigurement, and also greatest anesthesia, thus allowing the patient the least discomfort and giving the practitioner most time to proceed. Special attention must be paid to fixing the lip by traction when dermabrading the lip, which can be ensnared in the machine causing significant laceration. Staying constantly parallel to the surface is essential, especially in areas of complex curvature such as the chin and malar eminences. Dermabrasion should always be carried out within the facial cosmetic units to avoid demarcation by pigmentation when and if possible. Dermabrading to just beneath the jaw line, out to the preauricular area and up to the suborbital areas ensures that a uniform texture and appearance is achieved. Trichloracetic acid (35%) can be applied to any unabraded skin, the eyebrows, and the first few centimeters of the hairline, to further improve blending of pigmentation.

Immediately following the procedure, excessive bleeding is controlled by the application of topical thrombin. Pain relief is achieved as soon as biosynthetic dressings are applied at the end of the procedure. Postoperatively, patients are given prednisone 40 mg a day for 4 days, which greatly reduces postoperative edema and discomfort. One of the most important recent advances has been the use of acyclovir in patients who have had a history of herpes simplex virus. Begun 24 hours preoperatively at a dose of 400 mg three times daily and continued for 5 days, no patients on this regimen have developed postoperative herpes simplex, even if there was a pre-existing history of this problem.

Most patients re-epithelialize completely between 5 and 7 days postoperatively when biosynthetic dressings have been used. Some dressings (e.g. Vigilon) must be changed daily, whilst others (e.g. Omiderm) may be applied at the time of dermabrasion and left intact until they peel off spontaneously after about 5–7 days. Both of the biosynthetic dressings mentioned need to be covered with gauze held in place by flexible surgical netting. After the skin has re-epithelialized, the patients are usually restarted on topical tretinoin day 7 to 10 postoperatively. If the patient has a previous history of pigmentary problems such as melasma, topical hydroquinone is given at the same time as the tretinoin. If by day 10 to 14 the patient shows signs of disproportionate erythema, topical hydrocortisone (1%) is begun. Patients are cautioned prior to surgery that it will take at least 1 month for their skin to be normal in appearance. Most patients, however, are able to return to work within 7–10 days of surgery if light makeup is applied.

Complications

Milia are one of the most common complications of dermabrasion and usually appear 3-4 weeks postoperatively. If tretinoin is utilized postoperatively milia are rarely encountered, and when they do occur they usually respond quickly to tretinoin therapy. Acne flares are another common complication in patients who are prone to acne. If the patient has had active acne in proximity to the dermabrasion, the acne flare can often be prevented or treated by giving tetracycline in the immediate postoperative period. Although erythema is expected following dermabrasion, persistent or unusually severe erythema after 2–4 weeks should be treated aggressively with topical steroids to avoid scarring. Hyperpigmentation is avoided by daily use of a sunscreen as soon as healing has occurred and should be continued for several months. If hyperpigmentation begins to appear several weeks after surgery, the administration of topical hydroquinone and tretinoin cause its resolution. While infrequent, postoperative infection can occur as the result of dermabrasion. The most common organisms are *Staphylococcus aureus*, herpes simplex virus, and *Candida*. *Staphylococcus* infection usually manifests within 48–72 h of dermabrasion with unusual facial swelling and honey crusting as well as systemic symptoms such as fever. Herpes simplex infections frequently occur if the patient was not pretreated with acyclovir, and are recognized by severe disproportionate pain, usually 48–72 h postoperatively. *Candida* infections usually result in delayed healing and are recognized somewhat later (at 5–7 days), exudation and facial swelling being the clinical symptoms. Appropriate treatment with staphylocidal antibiotics, acyclovir, or ketoconazole usually results in resolution of the infections without sequelae.

References

1 Burke J, *Wire brush surgery*, Springfield, IL: Charles C. Thomas, 1956.

2 Mandy SH, Tretinoin in the pre and post operative management of dermabrasion, *J Am Acad Dermatol* (1986) 15: 878.

3 Hang VC, Lee JV, Zitelli JA, Hebda PA, Topical tretinoin and epithelial wound healing, *Arch Dermatol* (1989) 125: 65–9.

4 Maibach H, Rovee D, *Epidermal wound healing*, Chicago: Yearbook Medical Publishers, 1972.

5 Mandy SH, A new primary wound dressing made of polyethylene oxide gel, *J Dermatol Surg Oncol* (1983) 9: 153.

6 Alvarez OM, Mertz PM, Eaglestein WH, The effect of occlusive dressings on collagen synthesis in the superficial wounds, *J Surg Res* (1983) 35: 142.

7 Roenigk HH et al, Acne, retinoids and dermabrasions, *J Dermatol Surg Oncol* (1985) 11: 396.

8 Rubenstein R, Roenigk HH, Stegman SJ, Hanke CW, Isotretinoin, *J Am Acad Dermatol* (1986) 15: 280.

9 Moy R, Moy L, Zitelli J, Mandy S, Effects of systemic 13-*cis*-retinoic acid on

wound healing *in vivo* — *American Academy of Dermatology Annual Meeting*, 1987, Exhibit.

10 **Moy R, Zitelli J, Uitto J,** Effect of 13-*cis*-retinoic acid on dermal wound healing, *JID* (1987) **88**: 508 (Abstr.).

11 **Dzubow CM, Miller WH Jr,** The effect of 13-*cis*-retinoic acid on wound healing in dogs, *J Dermatol Surg Oncol* (1987) **13**: 265.

12 **Wentzell JM, Robinson JK, Wentzell JM Jr et al,** Physical properties of aerosols produced by dermabrasion, *Arch Dermatol* (1989) **125**: 1637–43.

13 **Field L,** Dermabrasion versus 5-fluorouracil in the management of actinic keratoses. In: Epstein I (ed). *Controversies in dermatology*, Philadelphia: W.B. Saunders, 1984, Chap. 8, pp. 62–102.

14 **Burke J, Marascalco J, Clark W,** Half-face planing of precancerous skin after five years, *Arch Dermatol* (1963) **88**: 140.

15 **Yarborough JM,** Dermabrasive surgery, state of the art. In: Millikan L (ed). *Clinics in dermatology, advances in surgery*, Philadelphia: Lippincott, 1987, Vol. 5, p. 75.

16 **Yarborough JM,** Dermabrasion by wire brush, *J Dermatol Surg Oncol* (1987) **13**: 610.

17 **Alt T,** Facial dermabrasion: advantages of the diamond fraise technique, *J Dermatol Surg Oncol* (1987) **13**: 618.

18 **Hanke CW, O'Brien JJ, Solow EB,** Laboratory evaluation of skin refrigerants used in dermabrasion, *J Dermatol Surg Oncol* (1985) **11**: 45–9.

19 **Dzubow LM,** Survey of refrigerant and surgical techniques used for facial dermabrasion, *J Am Acad Dermatol* (1985) **13**: 287–92.

20 **Hanke CW, Roenigk HH, Pinske JB,** Complications of dermabrasion resulting from excessively cold skin refrigeration, *J Dermatol Surg Oncol* (1985) **11**: 886–900.

18

Surgical treatment of hidradenitis

Leslie E. Hughes

Introduction

The surgical management of hidradenitis suppurativa is a complex subject for which no simple, straight-forward description is appropriate. The most difficult decisions relate to judging when surgery is appropriate and, if so, if the disease is severe enough to warrant radical excision. Medical therapy has not proved effective in our hands at any stage of the disease, but once deep subcutaneous sinuses have developed, the problem is a mechanical one. The pathology is now that of poorly drained sepsis rather than the primary process—perhaps androgen related—that under-lies hidradenitis. In our experience, once deep sepsis has developed most patients will eventually require radical excision, although this may not be indicated until the patient is fully convinced that a procedure of this magnitude is appropriate. Although only radical surgery will give long-term control, it is often better to temporize with lesser procedures until the patient makes this decision.

It is equally important to recognize that no case of hidradenitis is so severe or extensive that it cannot be relieved by surgery. Many patients are denied surgery on these grounds, but they should be referred to an experienced surgeon who is able and willing to undertake whatever procedures are necessary to relieve the condition.

Successful surgical management is completely dependent on detailed surgical technique, particularly in regard to the extent of excision. This is poorly described in the surgical litera-ture, so this chapter gives some empha-sis to surgical technique. Uneventful healing of these often massive wounds is dependent on specialized nursing skills and familiarity with the many minor hiccups which can occur during the healing process. These are learnt only through experience.

Choosing the patient who should have surgery

Surgery is indicated when hidradenitis interferes significantly with the patient's quality of life. When there are obvious deep sinuses with purulent discharge, there is little difficulty in recommending surgery. In cases of lesser severity, it is reasonable to recommend surgery to a patient who suffers a painful episode lasting on average 1 week every 2 months, and who has tried various conservative medical therapies.

It is a characteristic feature of hidradenitis that the lesions can come and go with remarkable rapidity, so that severe disease may look relatively benign a week later. Hence it is generally appropriate to accept the patient's account of the severity of the symptoms, even though the disease may look quiescent when examined. If there is any doubt, the patient should be asked to return during a flare-up. Similarly, if the disease regresses between being placed on the waiting list and admission, it is appropriate to proceed with surgery if the patient wishes it. If the patient's optimism at this improvement makes them reluctant, surgery should be postponed, although experience has shown that they will almost invariably return with severe disease and request surgery.

Thus patients should always make the decision regarding radical surgery themselves, but the dermatologist or surgeon must give them full information on the extent of surgery and postoperative morbidity. It is helpful for them to meet other patients who have had similar surgery. Likewise, it is helpful to have one nurse who takes a particular interest in the condition and who will act in a similar fashion to a mastectomy counsellor or a stoma therapist.

Surgical options

Surgical procedures can be divided into three types, local, conservative and radical. Local surgery (which may be by scalpel, diathermy, laser, etc.) removes one or more nodules with minimal surrounding tissue and is appropriate for small isolated lesions persisting at the same site. It can be performed under local anaesthesia and on an out-patient basis. The patient should be aware that it is palliative only—in a recent study of 72 patients, Jemec[1] found local control in only 15%. Nevertheless, 70% of the patients considered local excision to be more effective than the medical treatment modalities they had received. Jemec closed the wounds primarily. We prefer to allow the small wounds to granulate (the patient being taught self wound management) because it seems to be associated with less recurrence. Perhaps sutures initiate a further lesion by obstructing the duct of an adjacent apocrine gland.

Conservative surgery involves the excision *en bloc* of a group of lesions, but to a lesser extent than that required to remove all the apocrine bearing skin. It is appropriate where the patient is ambivalent about radical surgery, especially in the groins of young women where it avoids removal of the labia majora and mons pubis (Fig. 18.1). It is important that the patient is aware that new lesions may develop, since this will occur sooner or later in most cases.

Radical excisions are necessary to give a high chance of permanent control. They involve total removal of apocrine bearing skin of the region. This involves large areas and patients should be given a clear indication of what will be removed and the length and nature of the postoperative course. This is particularly important in the case of women with inguinoperineal disease, in view of the removal of the outer surface of the labia and the mons pubis.

Radical excision is recommended with confidence for axillary and perianal disease because morbidity is not great and recurrence is rare. Complete cure is not so certain with inguinoperineal disease and morbidity is greater, nevertheless most patients are well satisfied with excision because recurrences are more superficial and less painful than the original lesions. In contrast, recurrence is so common in the submammary region, even after wide excision, that we no longer practice radical excision in this region.

Management of specific sites

Axillary disease

It is perfectly satisfactory to operate on both axillae at the same time, although patients need reassurance that arm movement will not be greatly restricted during the healing phase. However, inguinoperineal and perianal excision are best done separately, as the surgical trauma of combining axillary excision with one of these is too great.

Extent of excision

This may be determined by demonstrating the extent of the apocrine glands by using the oxytocin/atropine/starch iodine test.[2] More commonly it is determined on empirical grounds. Where disease is severe and involves the whole dome of the axillae, it is cleared by 1 cm (Fig. 18.2). With lesser disease, the hair-bearing skin is cleared by 1 cm, with a classical anterior extension onto the anterior axillary fold. This extension is often indicated by an area of skin pigmentation. Lesser excision of more localized disease will result in a high incidence of recurrence, and so should be avoided. It is important that the excision extend no deeper than the axillary fascia, since this may lead to nerve damage and lymphatic obstruction.

Wound closure

While many techniques have been recommended, most are unsatisfactory. Adequate excision precludes primary closure, so primary closure is followed by a high recurrence rate.[3] The same is true of simple flaps, while larger fasciocutaneous flaps result in a bulky mass in the apex of the axilla, which patients find uncomfortable.

Skin grafting and open healing are the two satisfactory alternatives. Immediate grafting with meshed skin can achieve rapid healing in a proportion of cases but carries the disadvantages of an unsightly axilla and the discomfort and poor cosmesis of a donor site. Women particularly dislike these corollaries of skin grafting.

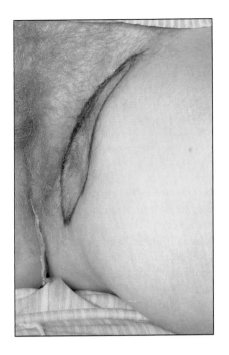

Figure 18.1

Conservative surgery indicated on the groin of a young woman.

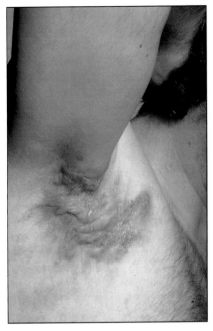

Figure 18.2

Severe disease involving the whole dome of the axilla.

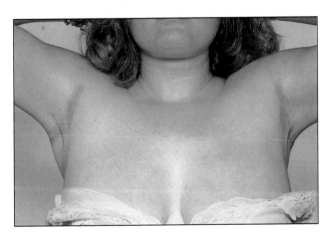

Figure 18.3

Healing by granulation after surgery to the axillae.

Healing by granulation has the advantages of predictable healing, a small inconspicuous scar and avoiding a donor site (Fig. 18.3). The functional results are equal and surprisingly good with both techniques. Likewise, hypertrophic scar formation, as sometimes seen in young patients, occurs with both techniques. The disadvantage of open healing is the longer convalescence, but in a randomized study of 10 patients undergoing bilateral axillary excision, seven preferred granulation, two preferred grafting and one disliked both techniques equally.[4] The superiority of healing by granulation has also been reported in the literature on plastic surgery.[5]

Inguinoperineal disease

The disease in this region may affect the hair-bearing skin of the suprapubic region, the skin of the inguinal groove (including the outer hair-bearing surface of the labia majora), the pigmented butterfly area of the adjacent thigh and the anterior half of the perineal skin. All this must be excised to give a high chance of long-term control. This formidable excision should be reserved for severe disease in well-informed patients. With less severe disease, local excisions are better used as a temporizing measure until the patient is convinced of the necessity for radical excision. Once the decision has been made, the full extent of skin should be removed. Less complete excision subjects the patient

to all the morbidity of a major procedure, but leaves them with later recurrence. In particular, leaving the skin of the labia majora is no kindness—recurrence in this site after a major skin excision is a devastating blow to a woman's morale.

Extent of excision

In women the extent of excision is as outlined above. The clitoris is carefully preserved by leaving at least 2 cm of adjacent skin. The external hair-bearing skin of the labia majora is removed but the inner aspect is carefully preserved. The butterfly area of the thigh is defined by the extent of pigmentation and the anterior half of the perineal skin included. Dissection should stay superficial to the fascia of scarpa (a depth of no more than 1 cm) to avoid damage to veins, nerves and lymphatics. The excision in a man is similar, leaving a 2 cm cuff of skin around the base of the penis and remaining superficial to the venous drainage superiorly. The scrotal skin is usually spared by primary disease, so a strip 1 cm adjacent to the inguinal groove is all that needs to be removed (Fig. 18.4).

Wound closure

These wounds are also best allowed to heal by granulation, even though this may take 3–4 months (Fig. 18.5). The slowest to heal is the butterfly area of the inner thigh, and we frequently take

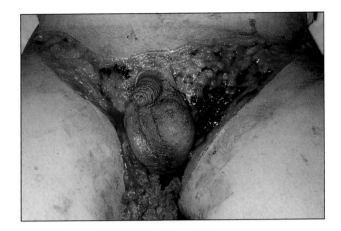

Figure 18.4

Extent of excision to the groin indicated for a male.

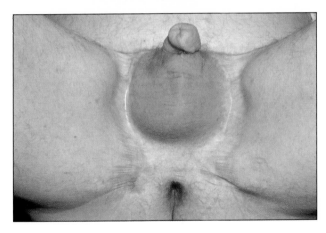

Figure 18.5

Healing by granulation after surgery to the groin.

a meshed graft from the excised skin, to avoid a donor site, and use it for partial cover of the butterfly area (Fig. 18.6).

Perianal disease

Perianal hidradenitis shows a surprising and not fully explained sex incidence of 10:1 in favour of men, whereas other sites show a marked predominance in women. Once established, it shows a marked tendency to progression, so surgery may be contemplated earlier than in other areas. Furthermore, the thickness and toughness of the buttock skin leads to widespread deep extensions in the buttock (Fig. 18.7). This is a further reason why surgery should not be delayed too long.

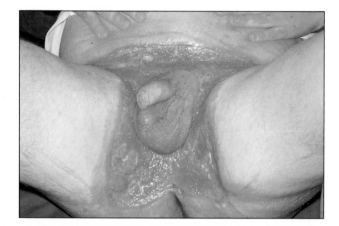

Figure 18.6

A meshed graft used for partial cover of the butterfly area of the inner thigh.

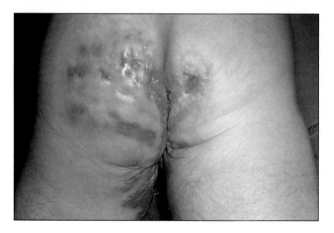

Figure 18.7

Widespread deep extension of perianal hidradenitis to the buttock.

Extent of excision

The apocrine bearing area of skin extends only about 8 cm laterally and posteriorly from the junction of the perianal and endoanal skin, and anteriorly involves the posterior half of the perineal skin. This is the extent of skin which requires removal in cases of normal severity. The anal canal is never involved primarily—apparent involvement is due to iatrogenic fistula or misdiagnosis such as with Crohn's disease. Thus the endoanal skin can always be preserved, and this avoids stricture formation or problems with continence.

In neglected cases, the buttock may become secondarily involved by subcutaneous spread. In these cases, once the perianal apocrine bearing skin has been removed, the peripheral extension can be managed by laying the sinuses open and curetting the granulation tissue. Only in the most advanced neglected cases does the buttock skin become so damaged that it must be excised and the defect grafted. The depth of excision includes only 0.5 cm of subcutaneous fat. In the region of the anus, skin only is removed to protect the anal sphincter and its nerve supply.

All advanced cases of hidradenitis are associated with marked vascularity, and bleeding is minimized by a diathermy excision. This is particularly so with extensive hidradenitis of the buttocks. Transfusion is often necessary, and in the most severe cases staged resection may be advisable.

Wound closure

The wounds heal well and relatively painlessly by granulation. As with other areas, healing is very much more comfortable if the wounds are dressed with silastic foam dressing.[6] The anal skin retracts out of sight at first, but reappears as wound contraction progresses. Skin grafting of this area is an unnecessarily complex approach. A proximal colostomy is never necessary. The wound need only be gently cleaned following defaecation.

Results

Wound healing

Wound management by granulation using silastic foam® dressings leads to predictable healing—slow at first but progressing rapidly as wound contraction develops. Wound healing takes 6–10 weeks for axillary and perianal wounds, and 12–20 weeks for inguinoperineal operations. There is surprisingly little pain during healing and patients are discharged after 8–10 days to continue their own wound care at home, with weekly clinic visits for supervision.

Delayed healing, pain and bleeding granulations are usually due to infection, this being staphylococcal in the axilla and anaerobic or mixed infections in inguinal and perianal regions. Infection is usually due to poor hygiene or friction from dressings which are too large or too firm in consistency.

Hypertrophic scars and functional results

Hypertrophic scars are unusual and are usually seen in young patients. Extreme scarring may interfere with final healing and require local excision. Later, scarring may cause limitation of movement. Most scars settle spontaneously, but a few require revision with a small skin graft or flap. However, it is important to recognize that further hypertrophic scar development may occur with secondary procedures, and also may be seen at the edges of skin grafts in susceptible individuals. Overall complications in 118 local excisions are given in Table 18.1. Skin graft failure is less common

Table 18.1 Complications following 118 radical excisions for hidradenitis suppurativa

Complication	No.
Early	
Skin grafting failure	9
Deep vein thrombosis	2
Anaemia	4
Local oedema	2
Late	
Hypertrophic scar	2
Wound pain	3
Restricted movement	3

Table 18.2 Recurrence following radical excision for hidradenitis

Site	No. of excisions	% Recurrence
Axilla	95	3
Inguinoperineal	41	37
Perianal	15	0
Presternal/ inframammary	6	50

now that meshed grafts are used routinely.

Healing by granulation rarely leads to limitation of movement either in the axillae or the groins.

Local recurrence

We have reported local recurrence rates in 82 patients undergoing radical procedures with a mean follow up of 4 years.[7] The results are given in Table 18.2. The results for axillary and perianal disease are excellent and reflect the well-defined and relatively small areas of skin which require excision.

The results of inguinoperineal excisions are less satisfactory, but better than appears on first reading. True recurrence is due to incomplete excision of the defined area of skin, most commonly the outer aspect of the labia or the posterior margin of the butterfly area. These may be cured by a further small excision or prevented by appropriate surgery at the primary procedure. A second form of recurrence is due to scattered lesions outside the standard apocrine area. These may be due to ectopic apocrine glands, or be more a manifestation of the tendency of these patients to acne conglobata. These scattered lesions may develop anywhere, and so cannot be prevented by increasing the extent of surgery. Fortunately, they are more superficial than the lesions of the standard hidradenitis areas, are less painful and can be treated by conservative measures.

Overall satisfaction

Of the 88 patients described above, 91% were sufficiently happy with the long-term outcome that they would wish to undergo the procedure again. Four of the eight remaining patients were dissatisfied because of local recurrence—a reflection of incomplete excision rather than of surgery *per se*. The remaining four were dissatisfied with their scars, although the appearance of the scars to a nursing observer was no different to those of the satisfied patients. It is of interest that one of these patients presented 4 years later requesting surgery for newly developed hidradenitis at a different site. When reminded that she had previously expressed dissatisfaction with the result of her surgery, she replied: 'I had forgotten how terrible is the pain associated with this condition'.

References

1 **Jemec GB**, Effect of localised surgical excision in hidradenitis suppurativa, *J Am Acad Dermatol* (1988) **18**: 1103–7.

2 **Morgan WP, Hughes LE**, The density and distribution of the apocrine glands in hidradenitis suppurativa, *Br J Surg* (1979) **66**: 853–6.

3 **Watson JD**, Hidradenitis suppurativa—a clinical review, *Br J Plast Surg* (1985) **38**: 567–9.

4 **Morgan WP, Harding KG, Hughes LE**, A comparison of skin grafting and healing by granulation following axillary excision for hidradenitis suppurativa, *Ann R Coll Surg Engl* (1983) **65**: 235–6.

5 **Silverberg B, Smoot CE, Landa SJ, Parsons RW**, Hidradenitis suppurativa: patient satisfaction with wound healing by secondary intention, *Plast Reconstruct Surg* (1987) **79**: 555–9.

6 **Morgan WP, Harding KG, Richardson G, Hughes LE**, The use of silastic foam dressing in the treatment of advanced hidradenitis suppurativa, *Br J Surg* (1980) **67**: 277–80.

7 **Harrison BJ, Mudge M, Hughes LE**, Recurrence after surgical treatment of hidradenitis suppurativa, *Br Med J* (1987) **294**: 487–9.

19

Electrosurgery and electrocautery in dermatology

Richard J. Motley

Introduction

Since the discovery of fire, heat has been used in the treatment of wounds. Neolithic skulls have been uncovered which show clear evidence of thermal cauterization, and records show that cautery was used for the treatment of ulcers and tumours of the breast from 3000 B.C. Hippocrates used heat to destroy skin tumours and his aphorism that 'heat will succeed where other methods fail' influenced medicine and surgery for centuries. In Medieval times, hot irons were used to control bleeding from battle wounds, and more recently it was not uncommon practice among pioneers to pour gunpowder into bullet wounds and ignite it to stem the bleeding.

The first electrocautery and electrosurgery machines were made 100 years ago and have contributed enormously to the development of modern surgery, yet despite their long association with medicine many dermatologists feel unfamiliar with the various machines and techniques available and do not employ these to their full potential.

Fire—a word of caution

Electrocautery and electrosurgery are both capable of igniting inflammable liquids and gases. Neither should be used in the presence of inflammable anaesthetic gases, and only aqueous antiseptic solutions should be used to clean wounds prior to surgery. Avoiding the use of spirit-based antiseptics will go a long way towards reducing the incidence of accidental burns. The element in electrocautery often collects tissue char which may need to be removed periodically during a procedure. A moist cotton swab should be available for this, as the heat from the element may be sufficient to ignite a dry swab. Care should also be exercised when replacing the cautery after use as undissipated heat from the element may be sufficient to burn equipment or other members of staff.

Electrocautery

The principal component of electrocautery equipment is the metal element or 'burner' which is heated by the passage of an electrical current. Elements are available in varying shapes and sizes according to requirements, and power is supplied by

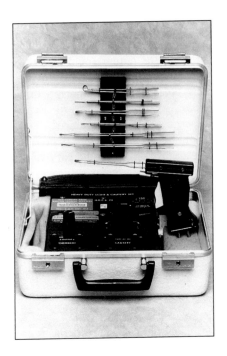

Figure 19.1

Heavy-duty electrocautery equipment. A variety of 'burners' are shown together with their handles (leads omitted for clarity).

batteries or a low-voltage transformer. The most durable electrocautery equipment is that primarily manufactured for cautery of the cervix; this has a heavy-duty element and requires a mains-powered transformer (Fig. 19.1). Portable battery-powered devices are convenient, but use fine and hence rather fragile elements.

Prior to use the element should be sterilized by heating to red heat. The voltage is then adjusted to maintain the desired temperature. Tissue destruction occurs through the physical transfer of heat and depends on the element's temperature and duration of application. These properties lead to a predictable level of tissue damage. No current flows through the patient and there is no risk of electrical shock or pacemaker interference.

Electrocautery may be used to secure haemostasis following superficial procedures and in combination with curettage for the destruction of skin tumours. In order to minimize fumes, the cautery element may be applied cold and heated up whilst constantly moving it over the tissue until the desired effect is achieved. Electrocautery is preferable to electrosurgery for treating lesions on the penis, and may be used on non-conductive tissue such as nail. There is scope for improving the design of electrocautery equipment and a temperature-controlled element would be a great advantage. Electrocautery is inexpensive, simple and safe to use, self-sterilizing, free of electrical risks and achieves predictable effects even in inexperienced hands. For these reasons a good quality electrocautery machine is indispensable to the dermatologist.

Electrosurgery

The heart of electrosurgical equipment is the oscillator or generator which produces a high-frequency electrical signal.

The application of direct current or low-frequency alternating current to the body causes muscle contraction and ventricular fibrillation at relatively low power. With increasing frequency, however, the threshold current for muscle stimulation rises and above 0.5 MHz sufficient power for electrosurgery can be delivered without muscle contraction or the risk of inducing ventricular fibrillation.

Unlike electrocautery, the heat of electrosurgery is generated within the tissues by the passage of electrical current and depends on current density. Current flows from the machine through the active electrode held by the surgeon, through the patient, and returns by way of a large dispersive patient return electrode. It is the path of this current flow which determines the safety and most of the hazards associated with electrosurgery.

Active electrodes have a small area of contact with the patient and this leads to a high current density and tissue destruction, whereas the dispersive patient return electrode has a large area of contact and minimal current density. Although the active electrode may become hot during use, this is insufficient to sterilize it and formal sterilization of the electrode between patients is mandatory.

The first electrosurgical generators consisted of a coil and capacitor connected in series with a spark gap. The voltage across the coil and capacitor rose until it was sufficient to spark across the gap, when a burst of high-frequency discharge occurred. This process repeated itself at 50 or 60 Hz, producing a series of discharges. The nature of the output could be varied by adjusting the spark gap to give more coagulating or more cutting effect. This type of spark gap electrosurgery generator produced good haemostasis, fulguration, desiccation and coagulation and would cut tissue if the available power was sufficient, but in doing so it created a considerable degree of lateral wound damage which prevented primary surgical repair.

In 1908, Lee de Forest (inventor of the vacuum tube) built a radiofrequency generator and asked Neil and Sternberger at Bellevue Hospital, New York, to try this on dogs. The oscillator produced excellent tissue cutting, but could not compete with spark-gap units for tissue coagulation and haemostasis. At that time the extent of lateral tissue damage adjacent to the vacuum tube oscillator incision was 0.1 mm compared with centimetres for the spark-gap machines.

With later development electrosurgical units were made which incorporated both spark-gap and vacuum tube oscillators and provided a choice of electrosurgical effects. Some modern electrosurgery units still employ this configuration, but increasingly these are being replaced by solid state transistorized units which can provide the same range of effects through internal modulation of their output.

The place of modern electrosurgery was really established by Bovie and Cushing in 1928. Bovie was a physicist at the Harvard Cancer Commission and had developed two electrosurgical units, one for coagulating and one for cutting. Harvey Cushing, one of the great pioneer neurosurgeons and the father of modern neurosurgery, had been concerned for some time with the problem of uncontrolled haemorrhage after hypophysectomy. In 1926, working with Bovie, he used electrosurgery to achieve haemostasis during the removal of a highly vascular cerebral tumour. The results were so impressive that Cushing called back many of his patients previously considered inoperable. Cushing and Bovie's paper describing their work was published in 1928.

Modes of electrosurgery

Monopolar electrosurgery is the application of electrical current to the patient through a single active electrode. A large dispersive patient return electrode may also be employed to direct the return current safely back to the machine.

Bipolar electrosurgery uses two electrodes either in the form of two separate but parallel needle electrodes, or as the two blades of insulated forceps. Current flows from one electrode to the other and only the intervening tissue is affected. No current flows through the body of the patient. A common misconception is that the use of surgical forceps to grip a bleeding vessel together with the application of an electrosurgical current from a monopolar electrode constitute

'bipolar' diathermy. Although the tissue held with the forceps is coagulated, the current is flowing in a monopolar fashion through the patient.

Electrosection

A continuous high-frequency current of at least 0.5 MHz delivered at high power through a needle-point electrode delivers the cutting action of electrosurgery. An intense electrical arc is struck between the needle point and the tissue. The continuous waveform and the pointed electrode serve to focus the arc which vaporizes the tissue, producing a scalpel-like cut.

It may surprise the inexperienced operator that virtually no haemostasis accompanies this mode of electrosurgery. There is, however, a considerable amount of smoke, and extraction facilities should be available to cope with this. Evidence suggests that viable viral particles may be contained within the plume generated by electrosectioning. Cutting and coagulating currents may be 'blended' to achieve a combined effect.

Coagulation, desiccation and fulguration

These electrosurgical effects are achieved through a more widespread dispersion of heat which is facilitated by intermittent electrical discharges—such as those produced by the original spark-gap generators. Coagulation occurs when current flows through a volume of tissue, raising its temperature sufficiently to coagulate the cellular proteins. This occurs in the tissue held between the blades of bipolar forceps or between bipolar needle electrodes. With monopolar techniques the electrode should be pressed firmly against, or inserted into, the lesion and the current maintained to produce this effect. The volume of tissue coagulated depends on the diameter of the needle, its depth of insertion, the current intensity and its duration. The larger the needle and the greater the depth of insertion the higher the current intensity and the greater the duration required to coagulate the tissue—a reflection of current density.

If a monopolar electrode is held against the surface of a tissue and current applied for only a brief period, dehydration of the superficial cells or 'desiccation' occurs. The electrode may be moved lightly over a tissue to desiccate its entire surface.

The monopolar electrode may be held slightly above the tissue and the output increased until sparks are generated—a technique known as 'fulguration'. The sparks (because of their highly focused point of contact with the tissue), cause cellular destruction, and the overall effect leads to superficial tissue destruction accompanied by charring of the tissue.

Electrosurgery and electrical safety

Unlike electrocautery and bipolar electrosurgery, monopolar electro-surgery involves the flow of electrical current through the body of the patient. The behaviour of the high-frequency currents employed in electrosurgery has much in common with radiowaves leading to sometimes unforeseen hazards. There are stringent safety codes governing the construction of electrosurgical equipment designed to minimize the risks, but it is still possible to cause accidental burns if the equipment is misused.

A detailed discussion of the physics of electrosurgical equipment construction is beyond the remit of this article, and for a full account the reader is referred to the excellent book by Pearce.[1] However, a few words of explanation of the more important points are justified.

The effect of electrosurgery is dependent on the current density at the active electrode. A large dispersive patient return electrode is applied to the patient to direct the electrosurgery current safely back to the machine. If this return electrode is in poor contact with the skin, the small area of contact will have a high current density and this may lead to burning from the return current.

Electrosurgery currents may 'leak' back to the machine by capacitative coupling without the need for a direct electrical connection. This characteristic is employed with low-power monopolar machines such as the Birtcher Hyfrecator. However, even with these machines, if a direct return path is established (e.g. by contact with a grounded lead) then the current density through this preferred route may be sufficient to cause a burn at the point of contact with the patient's skin. When not in the surgeon's hand the active electrode should be placed away from the patient, preferably in an insulated pouch where inadvertent activation of the unit will not cause injury.

Some machines use a capacitatively coupled patient return electrode. These electrodes are insulated from the patient and are applied loosely in contact with the skin, or just beneath the patient. This allows higher powers to be delivered to the skin and because of ease of use such electrodes have been popular in equipment primarily designed for dental surgery. The major disadvantage with this technique is that any breakdown in the insulation, or alternatively established point of direct contact with the patient's skin, may lead to a burn as the current flows more easily through a resistive rather than a capacitative route back to the machine. For this reason, direct contact patient return electrodes are preferred.

Most dermatology patients undergo cutaneous surgery with local anaesthesia and would immediately report any burning sensations from faulty return electrodes. It is the patient under general anaesthesia who is most at risk from faulty electrosurgical equipment or practices. Indeed, the patient under general anaesthesia may be attached to other pieces of electrical equipment for example an electrocardiographic monitor which must be compatible with the electrosurgery equipment.

The safety standards are designed to cope with these circumstances.

There is a situation in which inadvertent tissue damage may occur. If high powers are applied through a monopolar electrode to the distal part of a skin flap or to the tip of a digit or penis, all the return current must pass through the pedicle of the skin flap or the proximal part of the digit or penis and the current density, because of these anatomical restrictions, may be sufficient to cause proximal tissue damage. Bipolar electrosurgery and electrocautery are free of this risk and should be used in these circumstances.

The higher domestic mains supply in the UK and Europe of 220–240 V requires greater tolerances within electrosurgery generators than usually employed in equipment designed to run from a 110 V supply. For this reason some American machines may not meet European safety standards.

Electrosurgery and implanted cardiac pacemakers

The flow of electrosurgery current within patients with an implanted cardiac pacemaker may be misinterpreted by the device as a string of R waves, leading to inappropriate cessation of external pacing. Alternatively, the electrical circuits of the unit may be damaged or their function reprogrammed in an adverse way. Modern pacemakers are less susceptible to electrical interference; however, a few precautionary steps are advisable.

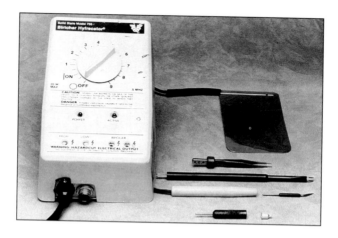

Figure 19.2

The Birtcher Hyfrecator. A single monopolar electrode is
commonly used with this machine for superficial tissue
destruction. Disposable sterile electrodes or an adaptor (shown
in the foreground) which allows the use of disposable metal
hub needles may also be used. Bipolar tissue coagulation may
be achieved with twin point electrodes and bipolar forceps
may be used for precise coagulation of bleeding vessels.
Although it is most commonly used without a patient return
electrode, its use allows the machine to achieve a more
powerful effect. (Leads omitted for clarity.)

Electrocautery or bipolar electrosurgery should be employed whenever
possible. If monopolar electrosurgery is
to be used the patient return electrode
should be sited in a position which
avoids current flow across the right
ventricle and short bursts of current
should be used. The main hazard arises
with urological diathermy which
employs the highest currents, and it is
unlikely that a problem would occur with
cutaneous surgery. The only safe course,
however, is to consult the patient's cardi-
ologist to obtain specific details about the
implanted pacemaker and to anticipate
some form of pacemaker interference
during the procedure.

Specific electrosurgery machines for the dermatologist

The Birtcher Hyfrecator

Within a decade of Cushing and
Bovie's paper, the Birtcher corporation

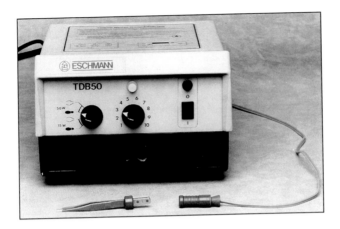

Figure 19.3

The Eschmann TBD50 bipolar electrosurgery unit. This unit is specifically designed for bipolar coagulation of blood vessels. It is used with insulated forceps and may be activated with a conventional footswitch or automatically when the forceps contact the tissue.

had produced the 'Hyfrecator', a low power spark-gap electrosurgery unit. Although the original design has been replaced with solid-state circuitry it remains the most popular form of electrosurgical equipment used by dermatologists (Fig. 19.2).

The Hyfrecator may be used for fulguration, desiccation and coagulation of tissue, but not for cutting. Used in the monopolar mode, a single active electrode is employed and capacitative coupling forms the return path. A bipolar output is available and may be used with bipolar forceps for haemostasis during surgery, with bipolar needle electrodes for localized coagulation, or with a monopolar electrode and a

patient return electrode for a more powerful effect. Sterile disposable monopolar electrode tips are available. The low output available from the Hyfrecator provides an additional margin of safety in its use.

The bipolar electrosurgical unit

There are a number of units available which are designed solely for bipolar tissue coagulation in conjunction with insulated forceps. The Eschmann TDB50 is one example (Fig. 19.3). These units allow fine, precise tissue coagulation and are used to achieve haemostasis during surgery. No

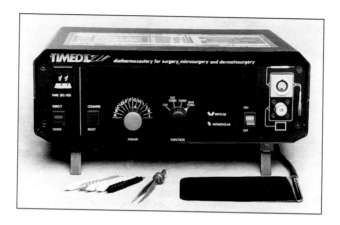

Figure 19.4

The Timed TD100 programmable electrosurgery unit. This
full function electrosurgery machine delivers all modalities of
electrosurgical treatment and, in the programmed mode,
delivers precisely timed electrosurgical pulses. It is used in
conjunction with a matched set of monopolar electrodes and
a patient return electrode. (Leads omitted for clarity.)

current flows through the patient, no
return electrode is required and there
is no electrical risk to the patient.

Compared with the bipolar output
from the Hyfrecator, these purpose-
built bipolar units have a more
controllable effect and achieve
haemostasis with less sparking and
tissue charring.

*Programmable full-function
electrosurgical equipment for the
dermatologist*

Most full-function electrosurgery units
are designed primarily for general
surgery, and whilst these can be used
in dermatology they offer few advantages. The cutting action of most
general electrosurgery units is
relatively crude. Recently, the Timed
TD100, a full function programmable
electrosurgery unit designed specifically for cutaneous surgery, has
become available.

The Timed TD100

This is a solid-state transistorized
electrosurgery unit operating at a
frequency of 1.75 MHz (Fig. 19.4). It
offers four different types of output—
cutting; a blend of cutting and coagulation; low impedance coagulation for
use with bipolar forceps and high

impedance coagulation for use with fine monopolar electrodes at the skin surface.

The output of up to 100 W may be continuous or delivered in pulses of 0.01–0.99 s duration with a counter recording the number of pulses delivered. As with other full function units, a patient return electrode is required except when the machine is used in the bipolar mode.

The machine is used in conjunction with a set of monopolar electrodes carefully matched to the electrosurgical output of the unit. This gives the dermatologist precise control over the type and degree of tissue destruction. Very fine cuts may be made with the needle electrodes, producing virtually no lateral tissue damage and allowing the wound to be repaired immediately. Timed pulses allow electrosurgery to proceed in a series of small controlled steps.

With this unit the dermatologist has complete control over electrosurgical treatment, enabling predictable and reproducible effects to be achieved. It is now possible to reproduce exactly the desired electrosurgical effect simply by selecting the electrode type and electrosurgical settings which have been previously determined to give optimal results for any procedure.

The introduction of a programmable electrosurgery machine is a major step forward for cutaneous electrosurgery, and we may expect to see an increase in the popularity of this type of treatment among dermatologists.

Conclusion

One hundred years after the introduction of electrocautery and electrosurgery these techniques form an indispensable part of modern dermatological practice.[2] Electrocautery remains safe, reliable and convenient, although there have been no recent developments in electrocautery equipment. Electrosurgery offers a greater range of techniques, and the introduction of programmable full function electrosurgery machines offers a new level of precision in cutaneous electrosurgery.

References

1 **Pearce JA**, *Electrosurgery*, Cambridge: Cambridge University Press, 1986.

2 **Sebben JE**, *Cutaneous electrosurgery*, Chicago: Year Book Medical Publishers, 1989.

20

New lasers for old diseases

John A. Cotterill

Introduction

There is now a wide range of lasers available for the treatment of dermatological problems (Table 20.1). It is important to remember, when thinking about setting up a laser unit, that no one laser will do everything, so initially a clear definition of the clinical aims must be made. Most clinicians are not in the happy position of having enough financial support to buy all the laser systems available when first establishing a unit. If the primary aim of the laser centre is to treat port wine stains, then a pulsed tunable dye laser system to treat vascular lesions could be the primary puchasing consideration. If the practitioner is more interested in dealing with general problems in dermatology or plastic surgery, then possibly a CO_2 laser, or a combilaser (CO_2 + neodymium-YAG laser), may be of particular use. If the primary aim is to treat tattoos, or possibly pigmented lesions, then a pulsed dye laser emitting at 510 nm, or a Q-switched ruby laser emitting at 694 nm, would be the most useful. If the primary interest of the physician is in the treatment of some types of skin malignancy, laser equipment emitting red laser light around 630 nm and designed to be used as part of photodynamic therapy would be indicated.

The optical properties of the target are vital in determining the type of laser therapy that may be utilized in the treatment of that target and also in determining the final outcome of treatment. It must be remembered, for instance, that there is no such thing as 'a port wine stain'. There is a wide clinical variation in colour and vessel size between one patient and another. As a generalization, a port wine stain in children is pink and easily compressible and anatomically consists of many small vessels less than 100 μm in diameter. A port wine stain in an adult may have similar characteristics, but with increasing age matures to become purple in colour, and very large, and at times cavernous, vessels develop. Many of the vessels present in such a mature, purple adult stain may be greater than 125 μm in diameter. Thus, a mature adult port wine stain has quite different optical properties to those usually present in a port wine stain in a child, and this explains why port wine stains in children often respond poorly to argon laser therapy.

Although significant amounts of light are taken up by haemoglobin at 514 nm, the argon laser is a so-called 'continuous wave laser' and, even with computerized hand-held micro-

Table 20.1 Lasers available for dermatological use

Laser	Wavelength (nm)	Colour
Argon laser[1]	488/514	Blue-green
Ruby laser	694	Red
Q-switched ruby laser	694	
Neodymium-YAG laser	1064	Invisible
Frequency-doubled neodymium-YAG laser	532	Green
Q-switched neodymium-YAG laser	1064	Invisible
Carbon dioxide (CO_2) laser	10 600	Invisible
Combilaser (CO_2 laser + neodymium-YAG laser)		Invisible
Pulsed tunable dye laser[2] for treating vascular lesions	585	Yellow/orange
Pulsed tunable dye laser for treating pigmentary lesions	510	Blue
Copper vapour laser	511/578	
Continuous wave dye laser[3]	577/585	Orange

processors, the shortest pulse width presently obtainable is 30 ms. However, most argon laser therapy is delivered in pulses of either 100 or even 200 ms. The heat generated by such a long pulse of energy, if applied to a port wine stain, rapidly diffuses out of the tiny blood vessels present in a child's port wine stain and damages surrounding tissues, ultimately producing a lot of scar tissue. This type of continuous laser therapy is much more suitable for the adult with large vessels where, if a pulsed dye system is used, with a pulse width of only 0.5 ms there is insufficient time for the heat generated even to reach the walls of the large blood vessels. On the other hand, a pulse width of 0.5 ms is much more relevant in the treatment of port wine stains in children, where the vessels are small and the pulse width is so short that thermal damage outside the blood vessels almost never occurs. Indeed, the histological appearance of a port wine stain after argon laser therapy and after pulsed tunable dye laser therapy is quite different. After argon laser therapy there is frank thermally induced necrosis of tissue, whereas the pulsed dye laser induces an acute vasculitis, with minimal changes in the surrounding tissues.

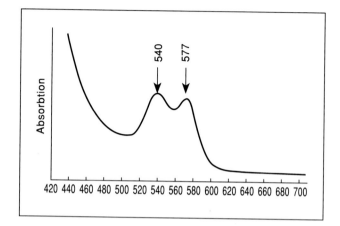

Figure 20.1

The absorption characteristics of oxyhaemoglobin.

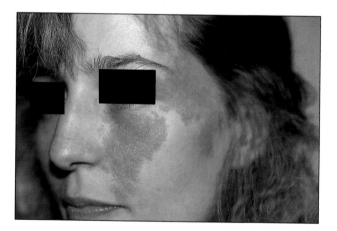

Figure 20.2

Port wine stain in young adult before treatment by pulsed tunable dye laser.

Figure 20.1 shows the absorption characteristics of haemoglobin. There are three main absorption peaks—at 415, 540 and 577 nm. It is not practical to treat lesions with 415 nm light because light at this wavelength penetrates skin very badly. This is partly due to the increased absorptive capacity of melanin for light of this wavelength.

Initially, pulsed dye lasers were constructed to emit light at 577 nm, but it soon became apparent that penetration of the lesion at this wavelength was not good. Penetration could be enhanced by a factor of 3 by altering the wavelength to 585 nm. Modern pulsed tunable dye lasers constructed to deal with port wine stains in children now all emit at 585

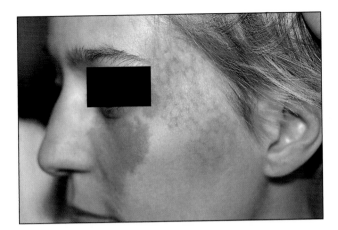

Figure 20.3

Port wine stain in young adult after treatment by pulsed tunable dye laser.

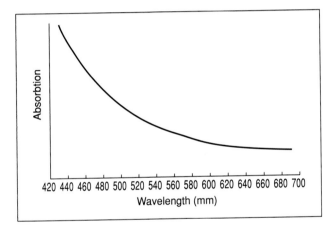

Figure 20.4

The absorption characteristics of melanin.

nm, with a pulse width of about 0.5 ms. The beam diameter is usually 0.3 or 0.5 cm and the usual energy fluence to treat patients lies between 5.5 and 10 J/cm² (Figs 20.3 and 20.4).

Pigmented lesions

Melanin absorbs well across the visible electromagnetic spectrum. Absorption is stronger towards the blue end of the visible spectrum and becomes progressively weaker with movement towards the red end of the visible spectrum (Fig. 20.4). However, there is sufficient absorption of light by melanin at the red end of the spectrum and this enables some pigmented lesions to be treated successfully by the Q-switched ruby laser, which emits at 694 nm.

Indian ink also absorbs well at this wavelength and this is why the Q-switched ruby laser is the treatment of choice for amateur Indian ink tattoos.[4]

It is also possible to treat both pigmented lesions and tattoos with a pulsed dye laser emitting blue light at 510 nm in very short nanosecond bursts, combined with an Alexandrite laser emitting red light. Both the Q-switched ruby laser and the blue pulsed dye/Alexandrite combined laser seem to work best on Indian ink tattoos. Treatment of some of the colours in tattoos may be difficult. For instance, the red areas in the tattoo usually do not respond well to treatment with the Q-switched ruby laser.

The combilaser

The combilaser consists of a CO_2 laser and a Nd-YAG laser, which can be used either separately or together. In addition, the Nd-YAG laser can be frequently-doubled to emit light at 532 nm. Thus, three separate laser modalities can be available in one laser unit.

It has been claimed that the major time factor in performing out-patient dermatological surgery is control of bleeding. Excision of lesions using the combilaser is claimed to reduce bleeding time considerably. In essence, the CO_2 laser is used to cut the skin and the Nd-YAG laser to coagulate blood vessels.

I feel that this sort of laser should be available in most District General Hospitals. This type of provision would enable interested dermatologists and plastic surgeons to undertake quite a wide range of different laser work, ranging from treating port wine stains in adults to a significant volume of dermatological surgery.

The frequency-doubled Nd-YAG laser, used in conjunction with a hand-held automated microprocessor, such as the Hexascan (see below) would enable the dermatologist or plastic surgeon to treat mature port wine stains in adults with the prospect of very good cosmetic results.

The hexascan[5]

There are several automated delivery systems now available. There is no doubt that these systems have revolutionized the cosmetic results obtainable with laser therapy. Thus, a Hexascan used in conjunction with either an argon laser or a frequency-doubled Nd-YAG laser of sufficient power will enable the pulse duration to be kept low (in the region of 30–50 ms). Such a short pulse duration ensures a high degree of patient acceptability, coupled with low tissue damage, so that the post-therapy crusting of the skin is minimized using the Hexascan.

The Hexascan is very well tolerated by patients, most of whom do not require any local anaesthesia for their laser therapy. The scanning device is also far less tiring to use for the operator and enables patients to be treated much more quickly than with hand-held laser techniques.

The copper vapour laser

The copper vapour laser emits blue-green light at 511 nm and orange light at 578 nm. The laser light emitted is in a quasi-continuous mode and effective pulse durations, therefore, are of the same order as those of the argon laser. The copper vapour laser may have an important part to play in the treatment of vascular lesions in future, in conjunction with scanning devices such as the Hexascan. However, far more powerful copper vapour lasers than are available at the present time will be needed.

The copper vapour laser is expensive to run and its main drawback is the long time it takes to warm up before it can be used. The laser also liberates a great deal of heat, which can make work with the copper vapour laser very uncomfortable during the summer months.

Photodynamic therapy

The vascular endothelium of tumours preferentially absorbs porphyrins and techniques have been devised, using a haematoporphyrin derivative (given usually parenterally or sometimes topically), to treat a wide variety of different tumours. If the haematoporphyrin derivative is given systemically the patient remains photosensitized for a considerable length of time and this may make therapy difficult during the summer months. However, photodynamic therapy seems to be an effective way of dealing with patients having the multiple lesions of Bowen's disease. The lesions are usually irradiated with a red laser light of around 630 nm wavelength derived from gold vapour or the continuous wave dye system. The procedure is quite painful for patients and some choose not to repeat the performance.

Conclusions

A bewildering array of lasers is now available to interested dermatologists and plastic surgeons. Technically it is possible to treat many lesions with lasers, but this should only be done if laser therapy is the best treatment available. For example, patients may be impressed if a mundane basal cell papilloma is removed with a CO_2 laser, but the ultimate cosmetic result would be far inferior to simple curettage. Laser technology is expanding at an ever-increasing pace and the prospects for its use by the next generation of dermatologists and plastic surgeons look very bright indeed.

References

1 Carruth JAS, Shakespeare T, Toward the ideal treatment for the port wine stain with the argon laser: better prediction and an 'optimal' technique, *Lasers Surg Med* (1986) 6: 2–4.

2 Tan OT, Sherwood K, Gilchrist BA, Treatment of children with port wine stains using the flashlamp-pulsed-tunable dye laser, *N Engl J Med* (1989) 320: 416–21.

3 Lanigan SW, Cartwright P, Cotterill JA, Continuous dye laser therapy of port wine stains, *Br J Dermatol* (1989) 121: 345–52.

4 Reid WH, Miller ID, Murphy IJ et al, Q-switched ruby laser treatment of tattoos: a nine-year experience, *Br J Plast Surg* (1990) 43: 663–9.

5   McDaniel DH, Mordon S, Hexascan: a new robotised scanning laser handpiece, *Cutis* (1990) 45: 300–5.

21

Intoxicated by port wine stains—the treatment of port wine stains with a pulsed tunable dye laser

Sean W. Lanigan

Introduction

Port wine stains are benign vascular naevi consisting of mature ectatic dermal blood vessels most of which are full of erythrocytes. There is a progressive dilatation of these vascular channels with ageing. These changes are associated with a colour change of the naevi from pink to purple.[1] Port wine stains affect 0.3% of newborns;[2] they occur most frequently on the face and persist throughout life, presenting a major psychological burden to the patient.[3]

Prior to the development of medical lasers in the mid-1960s, the treatment of port wine stains was generally unsuccessful. Treatment such as cryotherapy, irradiation and tattooing have been abandoned because of inconsistent results and scarring. Nowadays lasers such as the argon and dye lasers are considered the treatment of choice for vascular naevi and produce highly satisfactory results in the majority of patients. In this chapter I discuss the development of the pulsed tunable dye laser and its use in the treatment of port wine stains.

Argon laser

The argon laser was invented in 1964 by William Bridges. It was first used medically in the treatment of retinal disorders and subsequently cutaneous vascular lesions. There is over 20 years experience with the use of the argon laser in treatment of vascular naevi,[4] and this has been the most widely used laser world-wide.

The argon laser emits blue-green light, and 80% of this energy is at wavelengths of 488 and 514.5 nm. This light is preferentially absorbed by the red colour of haemoglobin and to a lesser extent the brown colour of melanin. The light energy is thus absorbed by the ectatic vessels within the superficial dermis of port wine stains. The absorbed light energy is converted to heat, which leads to red cell destruction and thrombosis of small blood vessels. Blood flow decreases and the blood vessels subsequently collapse. Larger and deeper vessels are spared, as are skin appendages, in particular hair follicles. This thermal reaction produces lightening of the skin due to a reduction in haemoglobin, but also some dermal scarring and contraction similar to a second-degree burn.

Treatment is usually performed under local or general anaesthesia as the laser beam imparts a burning or pricking sensation. The spot diameter of the laser beam on the skin is usually 1 mm, and using an individual pulse technique to treat a port wine stain on half the face would involve over 20 000 separate impulses and take several hours; this is tiring and time-consuming for both patient and physician. The development of robotized scanning devices[5] has made treatment of large areas considerably easier and quicker. Immediately following treatment an epidermal blister develops with weeping and crusting of the treated skin, this settles over 1–2 weeks. The effects of treatment take 4–6 months to become apparent, with a gradual lightening of the treated area developing. Full lightening of the treated area may take 12–18 months to develop. Most large series of treated patients suggest that good results can be expected in 60–80% of patients with port wine stains treated with the argon laser.[5–7] In general, an 'excellent' result indicates complete, or almost complete, replacement of the port wine stain by normal appearing skin. 'Good' results have less than total removal of the port wine stain with no scarring. Assessments are usually made in an entirely subjective manner.

Computer analysis of biopsies of port wine stains and clinical correlates has demonstrated that the best results from argon laser therapy are to be expected in patients with most red blood cells and dilated vessels within the port wine stain.[1] These patients are generally older with red or purple rather than pink port wine stains. This work has been confirmed in clinical practice where results are considerably better in adults compared with children.[8]

The major complications of argon laser therapy are scarring and pigmentary disturbances. Scarring may be hypertrophic or atrophic. Hypertrophic scarring is more problematic and can range from 0 to 26%.[8] In children this can rise to 40% and severely limits the use of this laser in this age group.

Yellow light lasers

In order to improve the selective absorption of laser light by cutaneous blood vessels, a number of lasers have been developed with wavelengths around 577 nm which coincides with an absorption peak of oxyhaemoglobin (Table 21.1). Light at this longer wavelength is also less well absorbed by melanin than argon laser wavelengths.

The argon pumped dye laser has a rhodamine dye activated by argon laser light to produce a continuous beam of light at 577 nm. Studies with this laser have demonstrated its value in the treatment of adults with port-wine stains.[9] The longer pulse durations achieved with this laser have limited its usefulness in children; attachment to a scanning device has shortened treatment times and may reduce scarring rates.[10]

Table 21.1 Yellow light lasers used in the treatment of port wine stains

Laser	Possible wavelength(s) (nm)	Pulse duration
Argon pumped dye	488, 514, 575–630	0.2 s to continuous
Flashlamp pumped dye	585	450 μs
Copper vapour	511, 578	25 ns at 15 kHz

Yellow light may also be produced by using a copper vapour laser. Unlike the dye laser systems, light emitting from this laser is a rapid train of short, low-energy pulses (25 ns pulses, 15 000 pulses/s) in contrast to a single high-energy pulse or continuous wave. Most of the experience in the treatment of port wine stains with this type of laser has been from Australia.[11,12] Results are similar to those with the argon and continuous-wave dye laser in that adult port wine stains respond well, and light pink port-wine stains in children do not. Scarring rates (3.5%[12]) are superior to those with the argon laser. A comparative study of the copper vapour laser and the pulsed tunable dye laser in the treatment of port wine stains showed that the latter laser is superior in terms of paling of the naevus and development of atrophic changes.[13]

Flashlamp pumped pulsed tunable dye laser

The flashlamp pulsed dye laser was developed in the 1980s. It was the first laser to deliberately incorporate those parameters necessary to selectively damage cutaneous blood vessels based on theoretical observations concerning the optical properties of skin. By careful choice of wavelength, pulse duration and energy density, thermal injury confined to targeted blood vessels can be achieved.[14]

This laser was initially used at a wavelength of 577 nm with a penetration depth of 0.5 mm below the dermal–epidermal junction. Preliminary studies revealed high response rates with minimal complications.[15] Although 577 nm coincides with an absorption peak of oxyhaemoglobin, by increasing the wavelength to 585 nm penetration depth is increased to 1.2 mm in port wine stain skin, whilst maintaining the same degree of vascular selectivity.[16] By using microsecond pulses it is possible to confine thermal injury to targeted blood vessels within the port wine stain, and histological studies have confirmed the selective vascular injury induced by this laser with minimal damage to the overlying epidermis.[17]

There is considerable clinical evidence for the benefits of the pulsed tunable dye laser in the treatment of vascular birthmarks.[18] Particularly advantageous is the very low risk of scarring with this laser and it is highly successful in the treatment of port wine stains in children — naevi which have responded poorly to the argon laser in the past. Treatment can be undertaken safely in infancy.[19]

The laser generates spots of light 5 mm in diameter with a pulse duration of 450 μs. Typical energies of 6–8 J/cm^2 are used. The laser produces a well-demarcated bruise at the site of impact on the port wine stain which persists for 7–10 days. In general, no blistering or weeping of the skin occurs as the epidermis remains intact. This has been confirmed by video microscopy studies.[20] Because of the larger spot size, treatment proceeds considerably faster than with an argon laser and a half-face port wine stain can be treated in 30–40 min. Treatment is repeated to the whole port wine stain at intervals of 6 weeks to 4 months. An average of 6.5 treatments is required to clear a childhood port wine stain;[18] adults with greater ectatic vascular involvement often require 10 or 12 treatments. Discomfort is minimal and EMLA cream has proved a valuable anaesthetic for adult treatments, although many children may require general anaesthesia and be treated as day cases.

This laser should be considered the treatment of choice for childhood port wine stains. No other laser currently has a comparable safety profile in this age group. In adults other lasers can be considered. There is probably not one ideal laser for all patients and a choice of lasers available at individual centres is preferred. The pulsed tunable dye laser is considerably more expensive than other lasers used in the treatment of port wine stains and, although results are excellent in a majority of patients, objective studies[13] comparing the available lasers are required for rational development of this form of therapy.

References

1 Noe JM, Barsky SH, Geer DE et al, Port-wine stains and the response of argon laser therapy: successful treatment and the predictive role of colour, age and biopsy, *Plast Reconstr Surg* (1980) **65**: 130–6.

2 Jacobs AH, Walton RG, The incidence of birthmarks in the neonate, *Paediatrics* (1976) **58**: 218–22.

3 Lanigan SW, Cotterill JA, Psychological disabilities amongst patients with port-wine stains, *Br J Dermatol* (1989) **121**: 209–15.

4 Goldman L, Rockwell JR, Laser reactions in living tissue. In: Goldman L, Rockwell JR (eds). *Lasers in medicine*, New York: Gordon and Breach, 1972, pp. 163–85.

5 Rotteleur G, Mordon S, Buys B et al, Robotized scanning laser handpiece for the treatment of port-wine stains and other angiodysplasias, *Lasers Surg Med* (1988) **8**: 283–7.

6 Dixon JA, Gilbertson JJ, Cutaneous laser therapy, *West J Med* (1985) **143**: 758–63.

7 Apfelberg DB, Maser MR, Lash H et al, The argon laser for cutaneous lesions, *J Am Med Assoc* (1981) **245**: 2073–5.

8 Dixon JA, Heuther S, Rotering R, Hypertrophic scarring in argon laser treatment of port wine stains, *Plast Reconstr Surg* (1984) **73**: 771–7.

9 Lanigan SW, Cartwright P, Cotterill JA, Continuous wave dye laser therapy of port-wine stains, *Br J Dermatol* (1989) **121**: 345–52.

10 McDaniel DH, Mordon S, Hexascan: a new robotized scanning laser handpiece, *Cutis* (1990) **45**: 300–5.

11 Walker EP, Butler PH, Pickering JW et al, Histology of port-wine stains after copper vapour laser treatment, *Br J Dermatol* (1989) **121**: 217–23.

12 Pickering JW, Butler PH, Ring BJ et al, Copper vapour laser treatment of port-wine stains: a patient questionnaire, *Laser Med Sci* (1990) **5**: 43–50.

13 Sheehan-Dare RA, Cotterill JA, Comparison of the copper vapour laser and the pulsed tunable dye laser in the treatment of port-wine stains, *Laser Med Sci* (1992) **7**: 286 (Abstr.).

14 Anderson RR, Parrish JA, Selective photothermolysis: precise microsurgery by selective absorption of pulsed radiation, *Science* (1983) **220**: 524–7.

15 Morelli JG, Tan OT, Garden J et al, Tunable dye laser [577 nm] treatment of port-wine stains, *Laser Surg Med* (1986) **6**: 94–9.

16 Tan OT, Murray S, Kurban AK, Action spectrum of vascular specific injury using pulsed irradiation, *J Invest Dermatol* (1989) **92**: 868–71.

17 Tan OT, Carney JM, Margolis R et al, Histologic responses of port-wine stains treated by argon, carbon dioxide and tunable dye lasers, *Arch Dermatol* (1986) **122**: 1016–22.

18 Lanigan SW, A review of the laser treatment of vascular naevi, *J Dermatol Treat* (1991) **2**: 113–16.

19 Ashinoff R, Geronemus RG, Flashlamp-pumped pulsed dye laser for port-wine stains in infancy: Earlier versus later treatment, *J Am Acad Dermatol* (1991) **24**: 467–72.

20 Motley RJ, Lanigan SW, Videomicroscopy studies of port-wine stains treated by pulsed tunable dye laser. *American Academy of Dermatology Annual Meeting*, Dallas, TX, 1991, Poster.

22

Laser therapy of vascular, benign pigmented lesions and tattoos

Nicholas J. Lowe

Laser treatment of vascular lesions

Introduction

Numerous therapeutic modalities have been used to treat port wine stains and cutaneous telangiectasia. These have included electrocautery, cryotherapy, as well as a variety of lasers. Until recently, the argon laser was the most popular laser used to treat cutaneous vascular anomalies.[1,2] However, argon laser therapy resulted in a 5–11% incidence of undesirable scarring.

The concept of selected photothermolysis was developed using flash lamp pumped dye lasers specific to erythrocyte oxyhemoglobin in the dilated blood vessels and with short pulse durations so that only targeted vascular tissues are heated, producing better results with a smaller chance of scarring.[3–7]

Laser and clinical experience

In recent studies of port wine stains and cutaneous telangiectasia, we compared the results obtained with a flash lamp pumped dye laser and an argon pumped tunable continuous wave dye laser coupled with a robotized handpiece.[8] Details of the lasers are given in Table 22.1. The results are summarized in Table 22.2. Both lasers were used at the same wavelength (585 nm) in order to determine their comparative efficacy.

Discussion

The flash lamp pumped dye laser proved to be a reliable and effective treatment for port wine stains and upper body telangiectasia. The argon pumped continuous wavelength dye laser gave results that were less reliable and also produced some degree of scarring, even when used with the robotized handpiece. The degree of early blanching with this laser did not always predict optimum outcome of the vascular lesions.

One consistent early side-effect when the flash pumped dye laser is used is purpura, lasting for 9–13 days. It is possible to offer camouflage make-up to the patient if so desired. A summary of the side-effects of laser treatment is given in Table 22.3.

Table 22.1   Details of the lasers used for vascular lesion treatment

	Flash lamp pumped dye laser (Candela SPTL-1)	*Argon pumped tunable dye laser*
Wavelength (nm)	585	585 (other wavelengths available 470–630 nm)
Pulse width*	450 µs (spot size 2, 3, or 5 mm)	Continuous Robotized Hexascan (3–13 mm)
Energy range	5.5–10 J/cm^2	10–25 J/cm^2 (Hexascan) 0.5–0.7 W (handpiece)

*With the Candela (a SPTL-1 laser for port wine stains) a 5 mm spot size was used. For telangiectasia either 2, 3, or 5 mm spot size handpieces were used, depending on the extent of the telangiectatic blood vessels.

Table 22.2   Results of vascular lesion therapy

		Result		
Lesion	*Laser*	*None or poor*	*Good*	*Excellent*
Port wine stain	Candela (*n*=70)	4	36	30
	Argon (*n*=34)	20	13	1
Telangiectasia	Candela (*n*=84)	2	14	68
	Argon (*n*=34)	14	16	4

Laser therapy of benign pigmented lesions and tattoos

Lasers and clinical experience

There are a variety of benign pigmented conditions that might respond to selected laser photothermolysis.[9,10] They include solar lentigo, benign pigmented nevi, café-au-lait lesions, melasma, nevus of Ota and tattoos. Other therapies used for these lesions have included cryotherapy, electrocautery, carbon dioxide, argon lasers, dermabrasion and chemical

Table 22.3   Side-effects of laser therapy of vascular lesions

Side-effect	Duration (days)	Patients (%)
Candela FPDL		
Purpura	9–13	100
Crusting/scabbing	5–10	60
Hyperpigmentation		5
Scarring		5
Argon dye laser		
Immediate blanching	1	100
Crusting/scabbing	5–8	60
Atrophic scarring		30
Hyperpigmentation		10

Table 22.4   Details of the lasers used to treat benign pigmented lesions and tattoos

	Q-switch ruby (spectrum)	*Flash lamp pumped pigmented lesion laser (Candela)*
Wavelength (nm)	694	510
Pulse width (μs)	28	300
Energy range (J/cm²)	Superficial lesions: 3–6 Deeper pigmented lesions and tattoos: 6–10	2–4

peels. All of these have potential problems of overtreatment leading to hypopigmentation, postinflammatory hyperpigmentation as well as undesirable scarring.

Recently, laser modifications have allowed pulsed lasers to be developed which have the ability to treat pigmented and tattoo lesions while minimizing the risk of potential scarring and other undesirable complications.[9,10] We report our experience using two different lasers: a flash lamp pumped dye laser tuned at 510 nm,

Table 22.5 Results of the laser treatment of benign pigmented lesions and tattoos

		Result		
		None or poor	*Good*	*Excellent or clear*
Solar lentigo	Q-switch ruby	1	1	28
	Candela	2	14	5
Benign pigmented nevi	Q-switch ruby	0	2	3
	Candela	11	2	0
Café-au-lait	Q-switch ruby	0	12	13
	Candela	5	2	2
Melasma	Q-switch ruby	0	20	2
	Candela	7	2	0
Nevus of Ota	Q-switch ruby	0	5	6
	Candela	4	0	0
Professional tattoos	Q-switch ruby	0	8	19
	Candela		Not treated	
Amateur tattoos	Q-switch ruby	0	0	20
	Candela		Not treated	

and a Q-switched ruby laser tuned at 694 nm. Details of these lasers are given in Table 22.4.

For most superficial benign pigmented lesions such as solar lentigo and pale café-au-lait lesions, the two lasers gave equivalent results over a 6-month period (see Table 22.5). It remains to be seen which laser gives the longer term improvement of these lesions. The 510 nm tuned Candela laser also produced frequent purpura, which probably correlates with its absorption within oxyhemoglobin. Some patients developed increased

pigmentation of café-au-lait lesions with this laser. There was no scarring observed after treatment with either of these lasers.

For darker, deeper or thicker lesions there was a clear advantage using the Q-switch ruby laser. This may be a result of the expected deeper dermal transmission of the 694 nm wavelength compared with the 510 nm radiation. Good results were achieved with the Q-switch ruby laser in benign pigmented nevi, solar lentigo, some café-au-lait lesions and nevus of Ota. The response of patients with nevus of Ota were good to excellent after 4–5 treatment sessions per area.

Blue, green and black tattoos improved significantly or cleared completely on treatment with the Q-switch ruby laser using laser energy of 7–10 J/cm². Amateur tattoos cleared in 1–3 treatments and professional tattoos in 4–5 treatments (see Table 22.5), these being fewer treatments than reported with older Q-switch ruby lasers.[11]

It is clearly of vital importance not to treat potentially malignant pigmented lesions. When there is any doubt regarding the nature of the lesions, skin biopsies should be performed prior to laser therapy.

These lasers, particularly the flash lamp pumped dye laser and Q-switch ruby laser, represent major therapeutic advances for the lesions discussed. Both lasers showed virtually no risk of scarring in contrast to older lasers and alternative treatment methods.

References

1 Apfelberg DB, Maser MR, Lash H, Rivers J, The argon laser for cutaneous lesions, *J Am Med Assoc* (1981) **245**: 207–37.

2 Cosman B, Experience in the argon laser therapy of port wine stains, *Plast Reconstr Surg* (1980) **65**: 119–29.

3 Garden JM, The pulsed dye laser: its use at 577 nm wavelength, *J Dermatol Surg Oncol* (1987) **13**: 134–8.

4 Anderson RR, Parrish JA, Selective photothermolysis: precise microsurgery by selective absorption of pulsed radiation, *Science* (1983) **220**: 524–7.

5 Morreli JG, Tunable dye laser (577 nm) treatment of port wine stains, *Laser Surg Med* (1986) **6**: 94–9.

6 Garden JM, The treatment of port wine stains by the pulsed dye laser, *Arch Dermatol* (1988) **124**: 889–96.

7 Lowe NJ, Behr KL, Fitzpatrick R, Flash lamp pumped dye laser for rosacea associated telangiectasis and erythema, *J Dermatol Surg Oncol* (1991) **1**: 523–5.

8 McDaniel DH, Mordons S, Hexascan — a new robotized scanning handpiece, *Cutis* (1990) **46**: 300–5.

9 Anderson RR, Parrish JA, Selective photothermolysis. Precise microsurgery by selective absorption of pulsed radiation, *Science* (1983) **220**: 524–7.

10 Tan OT, Treatment of superficial benign cutaneous pigmented lesions using pulsed irradiation, *Lasers Surg Med* (1990) **12** (Suppl. 2): Abstr. 215.

11 Taylor C, Gange RW, Dover JS et al, Treatment of tattoos by Q-switch ruby laser, *Arch Dermatol* (1990) **126**: 893–9.

23

Management of patients with difficult disease

Treatment of the difficult acne patient

William J. Cunliffe

Introduction

Acne should be one of the most rewarding chronic skin diseases to treat since there is a wide range of effective therapies for most patients. The aim of this chapter is to discuss the management of the difficult acne patient, but a brief account of the management of less severe cases is an essential prerequisite.

Although the precise mechanisms of acne are not known, there are four major aetiological factors involved in its development: an increased sebum excretion,[1] ductal hypercornification,[2] colonization of the duct with *Propionibacterium acnes*,[3] and production of inflammation.[4] Drug regimens which affect these aetiological factors improve acne, and drugs such as isotretinoin which affect all these factors have a greater effect on acne than do other modalities. To avoid repetition, Figs 23.1 to 23.3 summarize the mechanism of action of the various treatments.

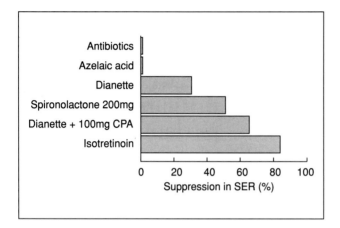

Figure 23.1

Effect of acne therapies on sebum excretion rate (SER).

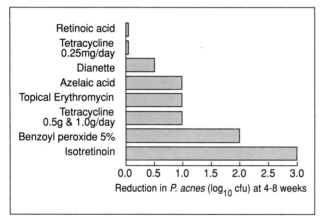

Figure 23.2

Effect of acne therapies on skin surface bacteria.

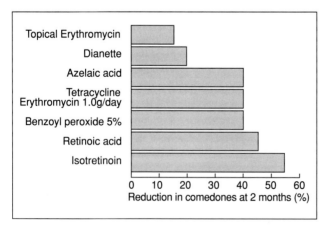

Figure 23.3

Effect of various acne therapies on comedones.

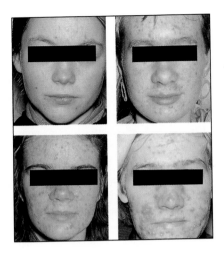

Figure 23.4

An example of an acne assessment. Assessments may vary from one doctor to another, but provided the doctor is consistent in his grading this is perfectly adequate.

Treatment approach

After the intial interview, decisions are made as to which treatment should be prescribed. The choice will depend on the severity, site and type of acne and its psychological and occupational effects. Some patients may have predominantly non-inflamed lesions, others may have more inflamed lesions, and in some patients there may be an equal mix of both lesion types.

It is important to emphasize to the patient at the outset the expected rate of progress. There is usually limited improvement in the first 2–4 weeks, but with the appropriate treatment most patients will see 40% improvement at the end of 2 months, 60% improvement at 4 months, and 80% or even greater improvement at 6 months. Total compliance is necessary. Failure to take the treatments correctly will markedly reduce the rate of response.

Clinical assessment

Ideally, any physician treating acne must use a grading scale (Fig. 23.4) to assess progress. Several simple subjective systems are available and are based on both inspection and palpation.[5,6] Some practice is necessary, but the benefits of learning such a system are immeasurable and instil confidence in the patients.

Uncomplicated acne

Mild uncomplicated acne

Subjects with mild acne (Fig. 23.5) should be assessed to determine whether the condition is predominantly inflammatory or non-inflammatory, or a mixture of these types of lesion. Subjects with predominantly non-inflammatory acne (Fig. 23.6) should be given topical retinoic acid,[7] isotretinoin or azelaic acid. This should be applied once or twice daily to all areas and, if appropriate, not just to the face but also to the back and chest.

If the patient has multiple inflamed lesions (Fig. 23.7) and very few non-

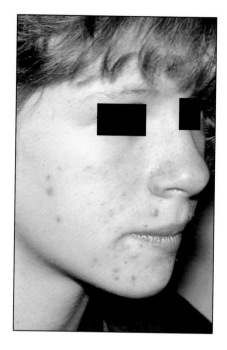

Figure 23.5

A patient with mild acne who should do well with topical therapy.

inflamed lesions, benzoylperoxide preparations,[8] topical antibiotics (clindamycin, erythromycin or tetracycline) and azelaic acid are all of help.[9-11] Despite many comparative studies, it is not easy to rank the benefits of topical antimicrobial therapy and adequate dose–response studies are lacking.

Some patients have mixed non-inflamed and inflamed lesions; such patients can be given topical retinoic acid, isotretinoin or azelaic acid in the morning and a benzoylperoxide preparation, a topical antibiotic or azelaic acid in the evening.

Moderate uncomplicated acne (Fig. 23.8)

A prospective study showed that subjects who received the equivalent of 1 g/day of tetracycline or erythromycin showed significantly greater improve-

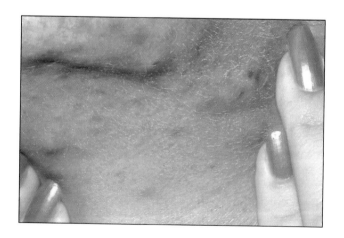

Figure 23.6

A patient who, on stretching the skin, has many non-inflamed lesions.

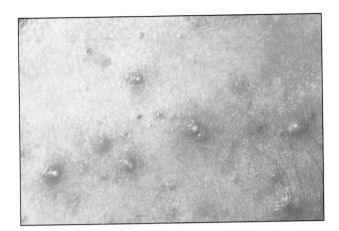

Figure 23.7

A patient with many inflamed lesions.

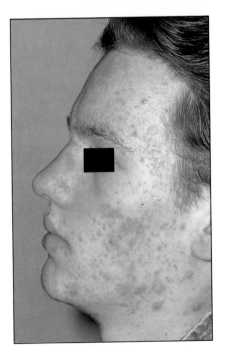

Figure 23.8

A patient with moderate acne who should do well with oral antibiotics plus appropriate topical therapy.

ment in their acne than those who took what used to be the recommended dosage of 0.5 g/day.[12] Furthermore, 12 months after stopping oral therapy, the rate of recurrence was significantly greater in those subjects who received the smaller dose. Therefore the conclusion is that the subject needing oral therapy should receive initially 1 g/day of tetracycline given as 500 mg twice daily. If after 3 months the patient is not better or worse, the oral therapy must be changed. The change should initially be to erythromycin or variants of tetracycline such as doxycycline and minocycline. We have considerable data to confirm the benefit of these therapies over tetracycline if the patient is not responding, but they are more costly. Erythromycin would be the drug of choice in women who may possibly become pregnant.[13] Trimethoprim is a further alternative but, before embarking upon yet another antibiotic, good microbiological control is necessary.

We have also recently demonstrated that patients who are taking the contraceptive pill should not take oral antibiotics because of the small but definite increased risk of contraceptive pill failure.[13] Thus, in sexually active women for whom there are no contraindications, Dianette (cyproterone acetate) ought to be given for 12 months in combination with topical therapy.

Severe but uncomplicated acne

Isotretinoin should be seriously considered in this group (Fig. 23.9).[14,15] Government regulations for the prescription of isotretinoin vary from country to country. For example, in the UK it is a hospital only, dermatologists only, prescribable therapy. Thus, government regulations and its cost may influence when and how it is prescribed. Different physicians use different regimens, but younger patients, especially men and those with truncal acne, do better on doses of 1 mg/kg;[16] other subgroups need only 0.5 mg/day.[17]

Patients with very severe acne often have cysts and in addition to isotretinoin, the resolution of the cysts can be aided by the use of intralesional triamcinolone or liquid nitrogen. If the lesion has been present for 10 days or less, triamcinolone is preferred; cryotherapy is preferred if the cyst has been present for longer. Triamcinolone works predominantly through anti-inflammatory mechanisms, whereas cryotherapy enhances

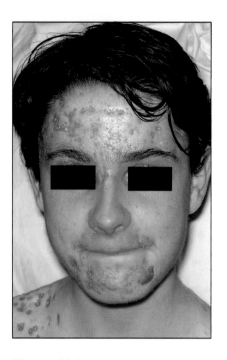

Figure 23.9

The patient with severe acne who should be given isotretinoin immediately at the first consultation.

the inflammatory reaction by breaking down the cyst wall and increasing defence mechanisms to come into play.

Complicated acne

Compliance is unquestionably the commonest reason for poor response. Even in a well-run clinic, lack of compliance, especially in less educated patients, is a major reason for poor response.

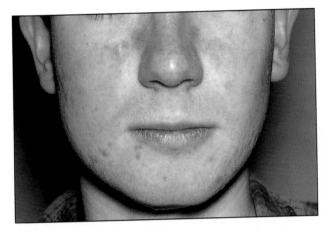

Figure 23.10

A patient with a typical primary irritant dermatitis associated with topical acne therapy.

Mild but difficult acne

There are several reasons for this clinical situation, which include an irritant dermatitis, acne excoriée, disproportionate depression, postinflammatory pigmentation and hyperpigmentation.

Primary irritant dermatitis

Virtually all topical treatments, if used excessively, will produce some erythema and some scaling (Fig. 23.10). This dermatitis is seen especially around the side of the neck and eyes. A moisturizing cream will help and, if the problem is excessive, a weak steroid ointment, such as flurandrenolone, will prove beneficial and resolve the dermatitis in a few days. The patient can then recommence with the same preparation but, if necessary, in a lower concentration and at a decreased frequency. Patch tests are rarely required.

Acne excoriée

Physicians tend to undertreat acne excoriée which may appear to them as a mild form of acne. Some patients in this group may not have acne but have a form of dermatitis artefacta, whilst some patients have relatively mild acne but cannot resist the intolerable need to pick at their spots. Oral therapy alone is required, however mild the problem; such patients do not usually tolerate physical therapy at all well. A sympathetic approach by the doctor is very important and in those patients who verge towards the diagnosis of artefact then pimozide (initially 1 mg/day) is indicated.

Dysmorphophobic patients

Many physicians are familiar with being faced with a patient complaining vociferously about his or her acne, yet

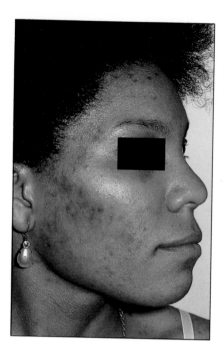

Figure 23.11

A patient with post-inflammatory pigmentation, a common feature of black skin.

therapy, even with oral antibiotics and, at times, with isotretinoin.[18] Their problem is to be considered seriously, as suicide from this disorder is not uncommon.

The professional patient

Most physicians are also familiar with the so-called 'professional patient', in constant contact with the public. Such patients are often doctors, lawyers, models or teachers and they are often very concerned about their appearance, no matter how mild the disorder. They are not psychologically disturbed; they simply wish to be rid of the spots. In such situations there is no point in trying to explain to the patient that his acne is really quite mild; they should be given oral antibiotics, and may have to stay on such therapy for a long time, perhaps for many years.

Hyperpigmentation

Subjects with black skin tend to develop hyperpigmented macules (Fig. 23.11). The severity of the pigmentation is not necessarily related to acne severity, so if a subject is developing pigmentary lesions, however mild the acne, it is essential that he or she be treated with oral therapy. Minocycline may occasionally produce pigmentation; this usually settles several months after the minocycline is withdrawn, but this side-effect is not necessarily an indication to stop therapy.

the physician has difficulty in seeing the spots, which are often of a psychological nature. Such patients need to be taken seriously and not asked 'Where are the spots?'. Neither should the patient be referred to a psychiatrist. Such patients may have a disturbed body image and usually a background of depressive illness; they are often obsessional. They usually have a monosymptomatic problem and it is necessary to treat the skin disease. Such patients merit aggressive

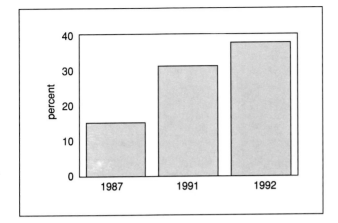

Figure 23.12

The increasing incidence of *P. acnes* resistance.

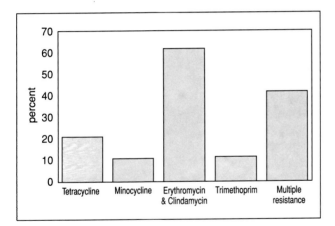

Figure 23.13

The individual antibiotic-resistant patterns in *P. acnes* resistant to antibiotics.

Moderate difficult acne

There are two major reasons why patients with moderate acne do not respond well to treatment: resistant bacteria and inadequate drug levels.

Resistant bacteria

Resistant *P. acnes* were uncommon but there is now an alarming increase in

Propionibacterium acnes strains resistant to antibiotics (Fig. 23.12). Figure 23.13 shows that resistance is mainly a problem with erythromycin, clindamycin and, less so, tetracycline.[19,20] Resistance to minocycline is rare. The assistance of an experienced microbiologist is necessary since *P. acnes* are not easy to grow. Swabs must be taken from the nose and the lesions to exclude Gram-negative folliculitis

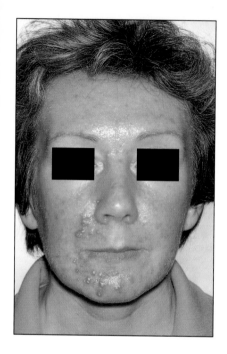

Figure 23.14

A patient with typical Gram-negative folliculitis; note many pustules.

(Fig. 23.14). In our department Gram-negative folliculitis accounts for 3% of our non-responding patients in this subgroup of difficult cases.

Working from these results the physician could then either treat the Gram-negative folliculitis or, if the *P. acnes* are resistant, use appropriate antibiotic therapy—minocycline is associated with a low level of resistance.[20] If the microbiologist fails to grow any Gram-negative bacteria and if the *P. acnes* are still sensitive then it

is quite likely that the reason for failure is inadequate levels of the drug reaching the pilosebaceous system.

Inadequate drug levels

Up to 66% of non-responding patients have a significant elevated sebum excretion rate;[19] this will produce a lower and ineffective concentration of the antibiotic in the duct. In this situation our therapeutic policy is to double the dose of the antibiotic or to use one of the brand-named antibiotics such as Minocycline (200 mg/day) or Doxycycline (200 mg/day).[21,22] Doses of 200 mg/day of minocycline produce serum levels which are usually above the MIC of *P. acnes* resistant to the minocycline. The addition of a non-steroidal anti-inflammatory, such as ibuprofen 400 mg twice daily could be tried in conjunction with the antibiotics for 12 weeks.

In non-responding women, hormone therapies may be appropriate, but investigations on the endocrine status are rarely required. Dianette is perhaps the most favoured therapy because of its ease of availability and relatively few side-effects.[23,24] It is important that the physician carefully manages the woman with respect to family planning counselling. If after 3 months the acne is still not improving, additional cyproterone acetate (50–100 mg/day) can be given from day 5 to 14 of her cycle because of its additional effect on suppressing sebum production. This regimen will usually

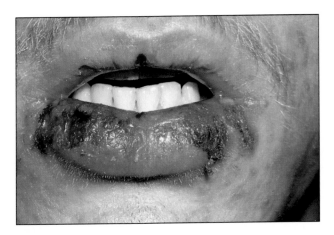

Figure 23.15

A patient with very severe cheilitis.

produce a satisfactory outcome, and after 6 months the additional cyproterone can be stopped.

If at any time the moderate acne is deteriorating and there is a risk of scarring, then isotretinoin must be given. Other indications for isotretinoin are in patients with moderate acne who have responded well on three occasions to conventional therapy but have quickly relapsed on stopping oral therapy.

Severe difficult acne

In most countries, most physicians will treat patients with severe acne with isotretinoin, but in some countries isotretinoin is not easily available and in other countries, such as the UK, it is budget limited and, despite its overall cost benefit,[25,26] there are financial limitations to prescribing it.

Nevertheless, in any patient with moderate or severe acne which is not responding well to conventional antibiotic regimens, ideally isotretinoin must be given. If isotretinoin is not available, alternative regimens include using megadose antibiotics, such as tetracycline or erythromycin (1.5–2 g/day) but this can be associated with gastrointestinal disturbance. Hormonal regimens such as Dianette plus cyproterone acetone (50–100 mg) from day 5 to 14 for 6 months can also be considered.

Some patients receiving isotretinoin do have complications; these may be predominantly due to side-effects or to poor response. The commonest side-effects are cheilitis (Fig. 23.15) and facial dermatitis. Up to 25% of subjects require medical advice for cracked lips or troublesome dermatitis, rhinitis sicca or blepharoconjunctivitis. Such patients may benefit from a medium strength steroid ointment such as flurandrenolone, often combined with the antiseptic clioquinol, and in extreme cases a swab should be taken and a relevant antibiotic given to eradicate the complicating *Staphylococcus aureus* infection. Some uncommon side-effects can produce marked problems such as the development of pyogenic granuloma. Single granulomas can be best treated with cautery, multiple granulomas with a potent topical steroid, such as clobetosol proprionate, combined with neomycin sulphate and nystatin twice daily. Multiple boils due to *S. aureus* infection may also occur and can be confused with resistance to therapy; in doubtful cases a swab should be taken and the appropriate antibiotic therapy given.

Of the systemic side-effects, teratogenicity is the most important issue and pregnancy must be totally avoided whilst on therapy and for 4 weeks after stopping therapy.[27] The commonest systemic clinical side-effects are arthralgia and headaches; usually simple therapies such as non-steroidal anti-inflammatory drugs (NSAIDs) or Panadol will control these problems but, as all side-effects are dose dependent a reduction of the dose may be advisable. If the dose has already been reduced, it is recommended that the patient be maintained on isotretinoin for 1–2 months longer, since relapse is more frequent if the cumulative dose of isotretinoin is less than 120 mg/kg.

Another complication in the management of severe acne with isotretinoin is a slow response. Up to 13% of subjects show a relatively poor response by 4 months, by which time most patients have responded well and need no further treatment. Close examination of slow responders will show (in 30%) multiple macrocomedones (whiteheads 1.5 mm or more in diameter). Isotretinoin will not affect these lesions which must be treated by alternative measures. Not only do they produce a slow response but are often a cause of quick relapse on stopping the isotretinoin. The treatment of choice for these patients is the application of the local anaesthetic EMLA for 90 min beneath polythene occlusion. On removing the polythene the EMLA is removed and the area touched gently with light cautery; this procedure ablates the macrocomedones satisfactorily.[28] The majority of slow responders do so for no obvious reason; but there is no cause for alarm as they will improve. A French group has also demonstrated that women who respond slowly have associated hormonal dysfunction such as polycystic ovarian syndrome, and this requires therapy with Dianette. The dose of isotretinoin is important with respect to relapse.

Severe but unusual acne variants

This is a very small group of patients with really difficult acne, but fortunately represents only a very small percentage of the difficult acne cases. In this group should be considered acne fulminans, pyoderma faciale and vasculitic acne.

Acne fulminans

This is characterized by the relatively sudden onset of systemic disease associated with moderate or severe acne, often in young males. The acne lesions are usually nodular–cystic along with papular, pustular and comedonal lesions, and often leads to scarring. The systemic features include fever, polyarthralgia, malaise, bone pain and joint pain. In addition, examination may reveal splenomegaly.

The reaction is without doubt an immune reaction to *P. acne* antigen and skin testing for *P. acne* antigen demonstrates a strong positive reaction at about 36 h, lasting for several days.

Although reported cases are few, it now seems fairly clear that isotretinoin should not be used initially but oral Prednisone (40–60 mg according to body weight) given over 6 weeks and gradually reduced over that time.

Therapy can also be started with tetracycline or minocycline in doses of 1 g or 100 mg, respectively, per day. Standard topical therapy for acne does not initially help much. What may be required is a topical steroid such as betamethasone valerate twice daily for the first 2 or 3 weeks. If after 6 weeks the acne is not responding the introduction of isotretinoin at a dose of 0.5 mg/kg per day can be given, but occasionally this can produce a flare in the systemic symptoms. The systemic symptoms usually respond well to oral steroids, and within a few days of starting therapy the patient feels much better.

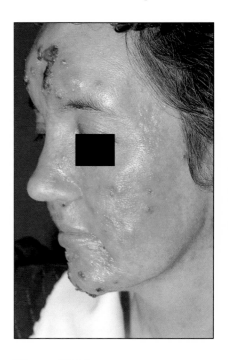

Figure 23.16

A patient who a few weeks prior had little or no acne suddenly developed very extensive pyoderma faciale.

A surprising feature of acne fulminans is that once the acne has cleared, even though the acne may return, the acne fulminans rarely recurs.

Pyoderma faciale

This mainly occurs in young women aged 20–35 years. It is characterized by the relatively explosive onset of central facial acne (Fig. 23.16), especially in women following a period of stress.

The patient is usually so psychologically devastated that hospitalization is often required.

Management is very similar to acne fulminans, but it may be possible if needed to introduce the isotretinoin perhaps a little earlier, maybe at the third or fourth week. As with acne fulminans, recurrence is very uncommon.

Vasculitic acne

This is extraordinarily rare; I only have personal experience of two cases. This is associated with pyoderma gangrenosum like lesions associated with deep pustular lesions and ulcerative lesions. In both patients the acne, prior to the onset of this event, was relatively mild. The end result is devastating because the scarring can be atrocious. Isotretinoin does not seem to benefit the patient, but therapy with azathioprine, prednisone and oral antibiotics such as minocycline and erythromycin seems to be the treatment of choice. Such cases should be treated as an acute medical urgency because of the sequel of horrendous scarring.

Conclusion

Space does not allow a discussion on acne scarring, but it is hoped that this review will permit doctors to better understand the ways in which acne should be treated. It is important that the dermatologist realizes that acne is a most treatable disease and this should be explained to the patient. There is no longer any justification for patients to suffer from acne vulgaris.

References

1 Cunliffe WJ, Shuster S, The pathogenesis of acne, *Lancet* (1969) i: 685–7.

2 Plewig G, Fulton JE, Kligman AM, Cellular dynamics of comedo formation in acne vulgaris, *Arch Dermatol Forsch* (1971) 242: 12–29.

3 Leyden JJ, McGinley KJ, Mills OH Jr et al, Age related changes in the resident bacterial flora of the human face, *J Invest Dermatol* (1975) 65: 379–81.

4 Norris JFB, Cunliffe WJ, A histological and immunocytochemical study of early acne lesions, *Br J Dermatol* (1988) 118: 651–9.

5 Burke BM, Cunliffe WJ, The assessment of acne vulgaris; the Leeds technique, *Br J Dermatol* (1984) 111: 83–92.

6 Michaelson G, Juhlin L, Vahlquist A, Effects of oral zinc and vitamin A in acne, *Arch Dermatol* (1977) 11: 31–6.

7 Fulton JE, Fazard-Bakshandeh A, Bradley S, Studies on the mechanism of action of topical benzoylperoxide and vitamin A in acne vulgaris, *J Cutan Pathol* (1974) 1: 191–200.

8 Fanta D, Clinical and experimental studies on the effects of benzoyl peroxide in the treatment of acne, *Hautarzt* (1978) 29: 481–6.

9 Dobson RL, Belknap BS, Topical erythromycin solution in acne, *J Am Acad Dermatol* (1980) 3: 478–82.

10 Becker LE, Bergstresser PR, Whiting DA et al, Topical clindamycin therapy for acne vulgaris, *Arch Dermatol* (1981) 117: 482–5.

11 Nazzaro-Porro M, Passi S, Picardo M et al, Beneficial effect of 15% azelaic cream on acne vulgaris. *Acne and related disorders: Proceedings of an International Symposium, Cardiff*, London: Martin Dunitz, 1988.

12 Cunliffe WJ, Evolution of a strategy for the treatment of acne, *J Am Acad Dermatol* (1987) 16: 591–9.

13 Hughes BR, Cunliffe WJ, Interactions between the oral contraceptive pill and antibiotics, *Br J Dermatol* (1990) 122: 5 (Letter).

14 Langner A, Wolska H, Fraczykowska M et al, 13-*cis*-Retinoic acid and tetracycline versus 13-*cis*-Retinoic acid alone in the treatment of nodulocystic acne, *Dermatologica* (1985) 170: 185–8.

15 Harms M, Masooye J, Radeff B, The relapses of cystic acne after isotretinoin treatment are age related: a long term follow up study, *Dermatologica* (1986) 172: 148–53.

16 Strauss JS, Rapini RP, Shalita AR et al, Isotretinoin therapy for acne; results of a multicenter dose response study, *J Am Acad Dermatol* (1984) 10: 490–6.

17 Hennes R, Mack A, Schell H et al, 13-*cis*-Retinoic acid in conglobata acne. A follow up study of 14 trial centres, *Arch Dermatol Res* (1984) 276: 209–15.

18 Macdonald Hull S, Cunliffe WJ, Hughes BR, Treatment of the depressed and dysmorphophobic acne patient, *Clin Exp Dermatol* (1991) 16: 210–11.

19 Eady AE, Cove JH, Holland KT, Cunliffe WJ, Erythromycin resistant

propionibacteria in antibiotic treated acne patients: association with therapeutic failure, *Br J Dermatol* (1989) 121: 51–7.

20 Eady AE, Cove JH, Holland KT, Cunliffe WJ, Superior antibacteria action and reduced incidence of bacterial resistance in minocycline compared to tetracycline-treated acne patients, *Br J. Dermatol* (1990) 122: 233–44.

21 Leyden JJ, Absorption of minocycline hydrochloride and tetracycline hydrochloride. Effect of food, milk and iron, *J Am Acad Dermatol* (1985) 12: 308–12.

22 Plewig G, Petrozzi J, Berendes U, Double-blind study of Doxycycline in acne vulgaris, *Arch Dermatol* (1970) 101: 435–8.

23 Aydinlik S, Lachnit-Fixson U, Lehnert J, Oestrogen-reduced ovulation inhibitors for the treatment of acne. Double-blind comparative study of Diane 35 and Diane, *Fortschr Med* (1986) 104: 547–50.

24 Carlborg L, Cyproterone acetate versus levongestrel combined with ethinyl estradiol in the treatment of acne, *Acta Obstet Gynecol Scand* (1986) 134 (Suppl.): 29–32.

25 Lafarge H, Levy E, Evaluation economique d'une innovation medicamenteuse: le traitment de l'acne severe par Roaccutane, *J Econom Med* (1987) T5(3): 117–27.

26 Cunliffe WJ, Gray JA, Macdonald Hull S et al, Cost effectiveness of isotretinoin, *J Dermatol Treat* (1991) 1: 285–8.

27 Rosa FW, Teratogenicity of isotretinoin, *Lancet* (1983) ii: 53.

28 Pepall L, Cosgrove M, Cunliffe WJ, Treatment of macrocomedones with EMLA, *Br J Dermatol* (1991) 125: 256–9.

24

Drug treatment of autoimmune blistering diseases

Louise Poskitt
Fenella Wojnarowska

Introduction

Bullous diseases cause considerable morbidity from widespread unsightly and painful erosions, blisters, mucosal discomfort and secondary infections. This group of diseases has a predilection for the elderly and our treatment regimens are very much influenced by the age of the patient. Drug adverse effects appear less well tolerated in this age group in whom many body systems ordinarily just coping, fail when the balance of one system is altered through drug therapy. As a group, they are invariably on other regular medications and become perplexed by changing regimens, e.g. alternate-day therapies. It behoves us to keep our regimens as simple as possible to facilitate compliance.

The majority of bullous diseases tend to improve spontaneously and, therefore, the *aim* of each visit should be to reduce treatment. Presence of minimal disease is not a contraindication to reducing systemic treatment but should be viewed as a measure that the patient is not being overtreated. Mucosal disease is much more difficult to control than cutaneous disease,[1] and often one may have to compromise by tolerating some mucosal discomfort in order to avoid long-term high-dose treatment. Secondary infection is often interpreted by patient and doctor as worsening disease activity, so a low threshold for swabbing and antimicrobial treatment is advised.

From our experience in the Oxford blister clinic, we have become much less rigid in which drug regimen we use for which disease. We now discuss individual drug treatments and then our management strategy for individual diseases.

Drug treatments

Glucocorticosteroids

Following the discovery of the immunological basis of pemphigus and pemphigoid in the 1960s, justification of their treatment with immunosuppressives was espoused. In 1979, Lever[2] advised high dose steroid regimens commencing at 180–360 mg to achieve rapid resolution of blistering eruptions. This was to be followed by a period of 6–10 weeks of daily high-dose prednisolone (to prevent relapse), before quickly reducing to 40 mg on alternate days with the addition of an immunosuppressant. Clearances were achieved in 38% at the cost of 9% mortality.[2]

Morbidity from prolonged corticosteroid therapy is now well known. Some of these are reversible such as psychiatric reactions, myopathy, hypertension, diabetes and moon facies.[3] Irreversible changes include posterior subcapsular cataracts, osteoporosis and aseptic bone necrosis.[3] In our experience, osteoporosis and oral *Candida* are the most troublesome.

Topical treatment is our starting point. Steroids can be applied directly to mucosal surfaces in the form of ointments (fewer excipients than creams) or via inhalers. Even with widespread bullous eruptions many patients are both clinically and symptomatically controlled with moderate to potent topical therapy (e.g. clobetasone propionate) alone. However, if after a few days to a week this proves to be insufficient, we commence prednisolone at 20–40 mg/day and increment at weekly intervals by 10–20 mg. The pursuit of complete blister abolition is not our aim, but rather patient comfort. We have found patience on the part of the physician pays! At these more moderate doses we avoid high-dose-associated adverse effects, e.g. psychosis, and yet we have not required any greater duration of steroid therapy in the long term.

Adjuvant therapy has a role in allowing prednisolone dose reduction and thereby reducing the attending steroid adverse effects. In the event of large doses, e.g. 60 mg, of prednisolone being required to control disease activity, we add an immunosuppressant, e.g. azathioprine, simultaneously, acknowledging that the latter may take 6–8 weeks for benefit to be accrued.

Dapsone

Dapsone monotherapy has been beneficial in 40% of our pemphigoid (both bullous and cicatricial) patients.[4] Cardiovascular disease, not uncommon in the elderly population, is aggravated by haemolysis and methaemoglobinaemia. We have seen angina and fatal myocardial infarction precipitated by dapsone. Haemolytic anaemia with dapsone therapy is universal and maximal at 4 weeks, but is dose related, as is methaemoglobinaemia. These can be catastrophic in glucose-6-phosphate dehydrogenase (G6PD) deficiency. Those with a racial predisposition for this should have their G6PD level checked prior to treatment. Cimetidine 400 mg three times daily reduces methaemoglobinaemia.[5]

We commence dapsone cautiously at 50 mg daily in the elderly, increasing the dose every 2–4 weeks (preferably 4 weeks) until control is achieved or side-effects intolerable. We assess full blood count and reticulocyte count weekly for the first 3 months (when these adverse effects are more likely, although they can occur at any time), and thereafter monthly. Usually there is a rise in mean cell volume with haemolysis, but a fall in this and the haemoglobin indicates iron deficiency which may occur in intravascular haemolysis. Iron parameters should then be assessed.

The most serious side-effects are agranulocytosis and hepatotoxicity which may occur in up to 1:3000.[6] Patients should be informed to seek medical attention if they develop a fever or feel unwell. Urgent full blood count and liver function tests are indicated as agranulocytosis and hepatotoxicity can occur at any time.[7] Dapsone hypersensitivity[8] and peripheral motor neuropathy are much rarer.[7]

It is recommended that women on dapsone who wish to conceive or are pregnant should take folic acid supplements. If possible, dapsone should be stopped predelivery in order to avoid the risks of neonatal haemolysis, hyperbilirubinaemia and methaemoglobinaemia. Dapsone is excreted in high concentration in breast milk and there has been a report of neonatal haemolysis in a breastfed infant.[9] These effects would be much worse in the presence of G6PD deficiency. We therefore feel obliged to advise our patients not to breastfeed, although this may be overcautious.

EMLA cream will increase the methaemoglobin.[10]

Sulphonamides

In a few patients in whom steroids have been contraindicated and dapsone not tolerated, we have seen a good response to the sulphonamides. Recognized potential hazards of sulphonamide therapy include neutropenia, agranulocytosis, hepatitis and severe cutaneous reactions, thus necessitating frequent full blood counts, especially during the first 3 months of therapy.[7] Haemolysis (severe in G6PD deficiency) and methaemoglobinaemia also occur with the sulphonamides. The same caveats in pregnancy and lactation apply as for dapsone. Obliterative bronchiolitis has been reported,[11] but because of the small numbers using this therapy it could be an underrecognized complication. Any complaint of breathlessness should be investigated. We usually use sulphamethoxypyridazine as it is better tolerated and potentially less nephrotoxic than sulphapyridine. We start at 250 mg and slowly increase to a maximum of 1.5 g. However, because the market for these drugs has been so small, drug licences have not been renewed in the UK.

Azathioprine

We have found this useful as a steroid adjuvant and sometimes as a steroid substitute in patients with poor steroid tolerance and uncontrolled disease. We advocate pretreatment (3 months weekly and thereafter monthly) full blood count and liver function tests to monitor for marrow suppression and hepatotoxicity.[7] Elderly patients, however, seem to tolerate azathioprine poorly because of gastrointestinal upset and we have had several cases of hepatitis.

Tetracycline and nicotinamide

This combination has been reported to successfully treat bullous pemphigoid and linear IgA disease.[12,13]

We have observed unequivocal reduction in mucosal discomfort in six of seven cicatricial pemphigoid patients treated with minocycline alone. Minocycline requires no blood monitoring and has few side-effects. Two of our seven patients, however, developed anterior shin hyperpigmentation and we wonder whether the elderly may be more prone to this than younger patients. We have seen a steroid-sparing effect of minocycline in pemphigus.

Methotrexate

This agent is not commonly used in the bullous diseases. We have treated three patients who have suffered from poorly controlled psoriasis and bullous pemphigoid. Both conditions have responded well to methotrexate in standard psoriasis doses. However, we would not advocate methotrexate routinely, as drug interactions and monitoring are major problems in the elderly.

Cyclosporin A

The role and dosage regimen for bullous disease is unclear. Anecdotal evidence suggests it may be useful as a last-resort agent.

Gold

Immunosuppressive gold therapy had a vogue in the late 1970s but failed to become established therapy as manifold side-effects, both dermatologic and systemic, failed to outweigh therapeutic benefit.[1] We have not had occasion to use gold.

Antimicrobials

We find *Candida* frequently complicates and exacerbates oral diseases and is mistaken for disease deterioration. We use systemic fluconazole.

Slowly healing erosions in bullous pemphigoid and pemphigus may be due to secondary infection. *Staphylococcus* is the commonest, but we have also seen *Pseudomonas* complicating scalp pemphigus. Our treatment is with combinations of povidone–iodine (Betadine) shampoo, topical silver sulphadiazine (Flamazine) and topical clobetasone propionate/neomycin sulphate/nystatin (Dermovate NN).

Disease management strategies

Pemphigus

First-line therapy is with topical clobetasone propionate and many patients manage with this alone. In those who do not, we use prednisolone in moderate doses, e.g. 30 mg, and rarely require doses up to 80 mg daily.

Steroid sparing can be achieved with use of azathioprine and/or minocycline. Anti-candidiasis therapy for oral and pharyngeal lesions is frequently required with systemic steroids.

Bullous pemphigoid

All patients are started on topical clobetasone propionate and this is all that is required by the majority of patients with localized disease. Second-line therapy involves dapsone or sulphamethoxypyridazine. If dapsone or sulphamethoxypyridazine prove ineffective, are contraindicated because of other concomitant medical problems, or the condition requires urgent treatment, we use prednisolone in moderate doses, e.g. 30 mg. Minocycline and nicotinamide are currently being assessed in a large trial in the USA. We have found azathioprine to be poorly tolerated. Review of Oxford patients suggested that mortality was increased in patients treated with azathioprine.[14] We have not improved on mortality figures compared with the pre-treatment era, but others have fared less well.[15]

Cicatrical pemphigoid

Topical steroids are first-line treatment followed by minocycline systemically. Dapsone or sulphamethoxypyridazine are then used if simpler therapies are insufficient. Prednisolone is then next employed and as a last resort, azathio-prine. Surgery is occasionally required for stricture release.

Pemphigoid gestationis

Some mothers can be managed with topical steroids, e.g. clobetasone propionate, alone. If not, then prednisolone in doses of 30–60 mg are employed. Should this fail then dapsone could be tried, bearing in mind the caveats described above. If both mother and baby are affected, pemphigoid gestationis in the baby usually spontaneously resolves within a few days.

Linear IgA disease

Usually dapsone or sulphamethoxypyridazine is our first line treatment. Those patients requiring other treatments because of drug side-effects seem to require high dose steroids, i.e. > 60 mg prednisolone. There are anecdotal reports or experience with using azathioprine, cyclosporine, minocycline and nicotinamide in linear IgA disease. We have found azathioprine helpful in two patients, but otherwise our experience with these other agents is limited.

In children with linear IgA disease we use dapsone 1 mg/kg, which usually means 25 mg on alternate days, and increase slowly if necessary. Occasionally, sulphamethoxypyridazine, prednisolone or topical clobetasone propionate are also required to gain better disease control.

Epidermolysis bullosa aquisita

Our experience with this disease is limited, but our few patients have been controlled on combinations of dapsone or sulphamethoxypyridazine, prednisolone or topical clobetasone propionate.

Dermatitis herpetiformis

Dapsone or sulphamethoxypyridazine are extraordinarily and rapidly effective in this condition. A gluten free diet is the preferred long-term treatment as it may reduce the risk of gastrointestinal lymphoma and patients feel better and gain weight on this diet. After 2–10 years of a gluten-free diet, dapsone may be completely withdrawn. It is rare to be able to reduce dapsone before 1 year.

It cannot be overemphasized that treatment should not be overenthusiastic in the elderly. There is no advantage in replacing disease death with iatrogenic death. Progress, in our view, is the development of greatest disease control with the fewest drugs and using those drugs with the least adverse effects.

References

1 Wojnarowska F, Briggman RA (eds), *Management of blistering diseases*, London: Chapman & Hall Medical, 1990, pp. 43–92.

2 Lever WF, Pemphigus and pemphigoid. A review of the advances since 1964, *J Am Acad Dermatol* (1979) 1: 2–31.

3 Truhan AP, Ahmed AR, Corticosteroids: a review with emphasis on complications of prolonged systemic therapy, *Ann Allergy* (1989) 62: 375–90.

4 Venning VA, Millard PR, Wojnarowska F, Dapsone as first line therapy for bullous pemphigoid, *Br J Dermatol* (1989) 120: 83–92.

5 Coleman MD, Tingle MD, Verbov JL et al, Cimetidine reduces dapsone-induced haematological toxicity in dermatitis herpetiformis (DH), *Br J Dermatol* (1992) 127: 426–7 (Abstr.).

6 Hornstein P, Keisu M, Wiholm BE, The incidence of agranulocytosis during treatment of dermatitis herpetiformis with dapsone as reported in Sweden, 1972 through 1988, *Arch Dermatol* (1990) 126: 919–22.

7 Wolverton SE, Monitoring for adverse effects from systemic drugs used in dermatology, *J Am Acad Dermatol* (1992) 26: 661–79.

8 Smith WCS, Are hypersensitivity reactions to dapsone becoming more frequent? *Lepr Rev* (1988) 59: 53–8.

9 Frayling IM, Addison CM, Chattergee K et al, Methaemoglobinaemia in children treated with prilocaine–lignocaine cream, *Br Med J* (1990) 310: 153–4.

10 Sanders SW, Zone JJ, Foltz RL et al, Hemolytic anemia induced by dapsone transmitted through breast milk, *Ann Int Med* (1982) 96: 465–6.

11 Porter JC, Friedland JS, Wojnarowska F et al, Alveolitis associated

with sulphamethoxypyridazine   (letter), *Thorax* (1989) **44**: 766–7.

12   Berk MA, Lorinez AL, The treatment of bullous pemphigoid with tetracycline and niacinamide. A preliminary report, *Arch Dermatol* (1986) **122**: 670–4.

13   Peoples D, Fievenson DP, Linear IgA bullous dermatosis: successful treatment with tetracycline and niacinamide, *J Am Acad Dermatol* (1992) **26**: 498–9.

14   Venning V, Wojnarowska F, Lack of predictive factors for the clinical course of bullous pemphigoid, *J Am Acad Dermatol* (1992) **26**: 585–9.

15   Bernard P, Venot J, Rommel A et al, Bullous pemphigoid: a prognostic study and review of 57 cases, *Semin Hop Paris* (1986) **62**: 1229–32.

25

Treatment of onychomycosis

Andrew Y. Finlay

Introduction

Onychomycosis is a very common problem; the recent introduction of several new forms of treatment make the management of this condition both challenging and perplexing for the clinician. In a recent survey, Roberts[1] demonstrated that the prevalence of onychomycosis in the UK was 2.8% for men and 2.6% for women. It is likely therefore that 1.5 million people in the UK are currently affected by fungal infection of the nails, the incidence of which increases with age.

There are several reasons why the management of onychomycosis is currently so confusing. First there are difficulties in making the diagnosis, as not all nail dystrophy is caused by dermatophyte infection. Second, it is difficult to decide whether or not a patient needs to be treated, as some patients are very disabled by nail disease whereas others have little resulting problems. Third, there are at least four different new drugs available

to treat these problems. Some clinicians still do not yet have a 'feel' for the confident use of these drugs or how to choose between them. Questions about specific indications, safety effectiveness, cost and instructions to be given to patients provide further confusion when several drugs with similar actions are introduced over a short time-span. Fourth there are problems for clinicians in judging the response of therapy because of the inherently slow growth of nail plate. Fifth, most new therapies have either been compared against placebo or against griseofulvin, and there are very few data directly comparing the new therapies.

It is therefore difficult to use any clear logic in planning therapy for a patient with onychomycosis. When the literature concerning new therapies is reviewed, the reader is left with the impression that every new therapy is significantly better than every other. This review will try to clarify each of the above main areas of difficulty.

Diagnostic pitfalls

Not every dystrophic abnormal nail is necessarily infected by a dermatophyte fungus. Indeed the commonest reason for failure of antifungal drugs is that the nail is not infected by a fungus in the first place. Both trauma and psoriasis are common causes of dystrophic nail. The changes in the nail plate in these situations may allow secondary invasion of other organisms, but unless the primary problem is dealt with treatment aimed at the secondary organisms will not result in significant clinical improvement. Dystrophic nails, from whatever cause, may also be secondarily invaded by various moulds; these include *Hendersonula toruloidea*, a grey-black mould, and *Scytalidium hyalinum*, a non-pigmented mould, both of which may be missed on culture of nail clippings. The brown spores of *Scopulariopsis brevicaulis* may give nail plate, especially affecting the big toe-nails, a cinnamon colour. *Aspergillus* species typically may affect several nails. Most of these moulds are resistant to the therapies that are usually used against dermatophytes.

The vast majority of fungal infections of nails are caused by dermatophytes, and in the UK it is unusual for *Candida* to be the prime cause of onychomycosis, though it is quite often detected as a secondary invader. There is some persisting controversy over the relative importance of *Candida* under these circumstances. One view is that if the primary dermatophyte infection is successfully treated the *Candida* will no longer be able to persist, whereas another view is that a drug should be chosen which will eradicate the *Candida* as well as the dermatophytes.

The most common dermatophyte infections are those caused by *Trichophyton rubrum* (85%) and *Trichophyton interdigitale* (another name for *T. mentagrophytes*) (12%): a few patients are infected by *Epidermophyton floccosum*. All of these organisms can produce distal and lateral subungal changes as well as total dystrophic changes. *T. interdigitale* may cause white superficial onychomycosis.

To treat, or not to treat?

Just because effective therapy is now available, it does not necessarily mean that all patients with onychomycosis must be treated. Every clinician will of course consider the benefit and potential risk to a patient before deciding on therapy. Points to note when weighing up this problem include taking account of the site of the infection, the degree of the patient's concern, and the potential long-term consequences of leaving the condition untreated. The site of onychomycosis is obviously of relevance as the handicap caused to most patients by having distorted finger-nails is much greater than the handicap caused by having abnormal toe-nails, which are usually covered. Abnormal finger-nails may cause problems at work, both because of interference with fine finger function and because of their adverse appearance. There may also be considerable discomfort around the nails in some patients with onychomycosis. The level of a patient's concern about their problem is obviously therefore relevant in taking decisions about therapy. When the long-term outlook is considered it should be remembered that not treating onychomycosis may result in further anatomical distortion of the nail and the nail bed. Untreated disease may act as a reservoir for recurrent dermatophyte infection of the feet, and for spread to other areas. Lack of treatment may also allow the possibility of secondary bacterial or candida infection which may become symptomatic.

Current drugs

Griseofulvin has been available for the treatment of onychomycosis for many years. This has now been joined by two topical agents, tioconazole and amorolfine, and by the systemic drug terbinafine. In addition, both itraconazole and fluconazole appear very promising for the treatment of onychomycosis but as yet do not have a product license in the UK for this indication. Key points for each drug are given in Table 25.1.

Griseofulvin is an inexpensive drug, but at best it only produces a 40% cure rate. Unfortunately, because it only has a fungistatic action, it must be taken over an extended period of time until all the infected nail has been shed. Considering that the drug has been available for over 30 years, it is disappointing that there are little or no *in vivo* data concerning the levels of drug that are reached in nail plate, and very little information concerning the penetration of griseofulvin through nail.

Terbinafine is very effective against dermatophyte infections and appears to have a fungicidal action. In a UK multicentre study,[2] patients with onychomycosis were treated for 12 weeks with terbinafine 250 mg/day. At follow-up there was a 82% mycological cure rate for toe-nail infections and a 71% cure rate for finger-nail infections. We have described[3] the pharmacokinetics of terbinafine in nail plate, and have demonstrated[4] that terbinafine when taken orally is rapidly detectable both in proximal and in distal nail plate in fungicidal concentrations. In an intriguing letter to *The Lancet*, Schuster and Munro[5] have stated that, although it is outside the recommendations, giving 1000 mg of terbinafine on only three occasions at weekly intervals can result in clinical and mycological response in patients with onychomycosis.

Tioconazole, as a solution applied twice daily, has been shown to be of benefit in improving the cure rate of patients taking griseofulvin. In one study,[6] patients taking griseofulvin alone had a 41% cure rate, but those patients taking griseofulvin with additional tioconazole being applied reached a 69% cure rate. The evidence concerning the value of tioconazole alone is, however, less strong.

Whereas tioconazole should be applied twice daily, amorolfine as a 5% nail lacquer has the major advantage of only needing to be applied once weekly. There is good evidence from *in vivo* work[7] that this drug penetrates nail plate at a rate of 20–100 mg/cm^2 per hour. In a study[8] comparing once weekly with twice weekly use there appeared to be some slight benefit in cure rate resulting from the twice weekly application, but this difference

Table 25.1 Comparison of drugs in toe-nail onychomycosis

	Griseofulvin	Terbinafine	Tioconazole	Amorolfine	Itraconazole
Indications	Dermatophytes	Dermatophytes	Dermatophytes	Dermatophytes, yeasts, moulds	No product licence: dermatophytes, *Candida*
Safety	Contraindications: severe liver disease; systemic lupus erythematosus; anticoagulants; barbiturates; oral contraceptives; headache; nausea; photosensitivity	Contraindications: severe liver dysfunction; impaired renal function; nausea; gastrointestinal disturbances	(Local irritation)	(Slight burning sensation)	Contraindications: history of liver disease; rifampicin, H$_2$ antagonists; cyclosporin; nausea
Nail penetration	No *in vivo* data	Rapid penetration *in vivo*	Data poor	Good *in vitro* evidence	Good *in vivo* data
Effectiveness	40% cure, 18 months	82% cure, 12 weeks	Improves griseofulvin cure rate	66% improvement or cure, 6 months	
Instructions	1 g/day for 18 months	250 mg/day for 12 weeks	Twice daily for 6–12 months topical	Once weekly for 9–12 months topical	100 mg/day (current maximum 1 month)

did not reach statistical significance. As well as its ease of use, amorolfine has the significant advantage of being active against some yeasts and moulds. It should be noted, however, that most patients with onychomycosis also have an associated fungal infection of the interdigital space or surrounding skin on the feet, and if a topical nail preparation is used it is necessary to also use a topical cream preparation to the surrounding skin, to try to reduce the likelihood of later reinfection.

Although onychomycosis is not a licensed indication for the use of itraconazole currently in the UK, this drug seems to have considerable potential for onychomycosis. It is effective both against dermatophytes and against *Candida*, and there is good evidence[9] that it penetrates the nail plate rapidly via both the nail matrix and the nail bed. Rongioletti et al[10] have recorded a 70% cure rate in patients with toe-nail infections and a 54% cure rate in patients with finger-nail infections using itraconazole 100 mg/day for 4–6 months.

Response assessment

When following up patients being treated for onychomycosis, response can be assessed both clinically and mycologically. From the patients' point of view, treatment will not have worked until they have normal nails. When griseofulvin was the only available drug, this therapy had to be taken over a full 18-month period while the nail plate was renewed. However, with the advent of drugs which both penetrate nail and kill fungi more effectively, it is possible to give a drug for a much shorter length of time, kill off the fungus, stop the therapy, and then wait for the normal nail to gradually replace the dystrophic nail which contains the dead fungal remnants. It is impossible to assess the clinical response of onychomycosis to therapy in a short time. Even the most effective treatment will take at least 10–12 weeks before a band of normal nail starts to become clinically apparent.

When mycological examination is used to assess the effectiveness of therapy it is important to bear in mind the mode of action of the drugs being used in order to interpret the results. If a drug which is fungistatic is being used, such as griseofulvin, nail clippings which are microscopy 'positive' indicate that the fungus is still present and may become reactivated if the drug is stopped. If, however, a fungicidal drug such as terbinafine is being used, clippings which are microscopy 'positive' may simply be clippings containing dead fungus and so the interpretation of direct microscopy is difficult and does not provide clinically relevant and useful information. The result, however, of culturing the nail clippings remains very important. If the culture is negative on repeated scrapings it is likely that the fungus has been successfully killed off, even though it may not yet have been fully eradicated from the slow growing nail plate.

A simple guide to therapy

In the absence of appropriate studies comparing the different modalities of therapy, decisions taken about which treatment to use may be largely arbitrary. However, the different side-effects and action profiles of the various drugs available make it possible to suggest a possible plan of action.

Initial patient assessment

When a patient with possible onychomycosis is first seen, the question of whether or not that patient should be treated can be addressed by assessing the site infected, assessing the degree of patient concern, and considering the long-term outlook in that patient. The risk factors for possible systemic therapy should also be considered for that particular patient. Clippings should be taken from the affected nails for mycology, in order to confirm the diagnosis.

First follow-up assessment

When the patient is reviewed with the results of the mycology, decisions will need to be taken about therapy. If the problem is primarily a dermatophyte infection and there is also widespread obvious associated skin infection, the use of terbinafine should be considered to try to eradicate the fungus both from the nail plate and from the skin. However, it should be noted that in onychomycosis terbinafine is only effective against dermatophytes. If yeasts and moulds are noted, the use of topical amorolfine should be considered. If *Candida* is present in the clippings the possibility of using itraconazole should be considered, though it must be noted that this drug does not currently have onychomycosis as a licensed indication. If there is a dermatophyte infection of the nail plate with very little associated skin involvement, and provided there is no specific reason why systemic therapy should not be used, then the question of patient preference between topical and systemic therapy has to be considered. If the patient prefers topical therapy amorolfine could be used, whereas if the patient prefers systemic therapy terbinafine would be appropriate.

Conclusion

After many years of relative slumber the whole area of treatment for onychomycosis is awakening. The availability of several new and effective drugs for the treatment of this very common condition provides a range of additional challenges for the practicing clinician. Successful patient management will depend, as always, on the basic fundamentals of good medicine, making a correct diagnosis and taking into account the risk/benefit ratio for any treatment that is considered. First, do no harm!

References

1 **Roberts DT,** Prevalence of dermatophyte onychomycosis in the United Kingdom: results of an omnibus survey, *Br J Dermatol* (1992) **126** (Suppl. 39): 23–7.

2 **Goodfield MJD,** Short-duration therapy: therapy with terbinafine for dermatophyte onychomycosis: a multicentre trial, *Br J Dermatol* (1992) **126** (Suppl. 39): 33–5.

3 **Finlay AY, Lever L, Thomas R, Dykes PJ,** Nail matrix kinetics of oral terbinafine in onychomycosis and normal nails, *J Dermatol Treat* (1990) **1** (Suppl. 2): 51–3.

4 **Finlay AY,** Pharmacokinetics of terbinafine in the nail, *Br J Dermatol* (1992) **126** (Suppl. 39): 28–32.

5 **Shuster S, Munro CS,** Single dose treatment of fungal nail disease, *Lancet* (1992) **339:** 1066 (Letter).

6 **Hay RJ, Roberts DT, Doherty VR et al,** The topical treatment of onychomycosis using a new combined urea/imadazole preparation, *Clin Exp Dermatol* (1988) **13:** 164–7.

7 **Franz TJ,** Absorption of amorolfine through human nail, *Dermatology* (1992) **184** (Suppl. 1): 18–20.

8 **Reinel D,** Topical treatment of onychomycosis with amorolfine 5% nail lacquer: comparative efficacy and tolerability of once and twice weekly use, *Dermatology* (1992) **184** (Suppl. 1): 21–4.

9 **Matthieu L, de Doncker P, Cauwenbergh C et al,** Itraconazole penetrates the nail via the nail matrix and the nail bed — an investigation in onychomycosis, *Clin Exp Dermatol* (1991) **16:** 374–6.

10 **Rongioletti F, Robert E, Tripodi S, Persi A,** Treatment of onychomycosis with itraconazole, *J Dermatol Treat* (1992) **2:** 145–6.

Index